$29 billic
Reasons to Lie about
Cholesterol

Making profit by turning healthy people into patients

$29 billion
Reasons to Lie about
Cholesterol

Making profit
by turning healthy people
into patients

Justin Smith

Matador
9 De Montfort Mews
Leicester LE1 7FW, UK
Tel: (+44) 116 255 9311 / 9312
Email: books@troubador.co.uk
Web: www.troubador.co.uk/matador

ISBN 978-1848760-714

A Cataloguing-in-Publication (CIP) catalogue record for this book
is available from the British Library.

Typeset in 11pt Book Antiqua by Troubador Publishing Ltd, Leicester, UK
Printed and bound in the UK by TJ International Ltd, Padstow, Cornwall

Matador is an imprint of Troubador Publishing Ltd

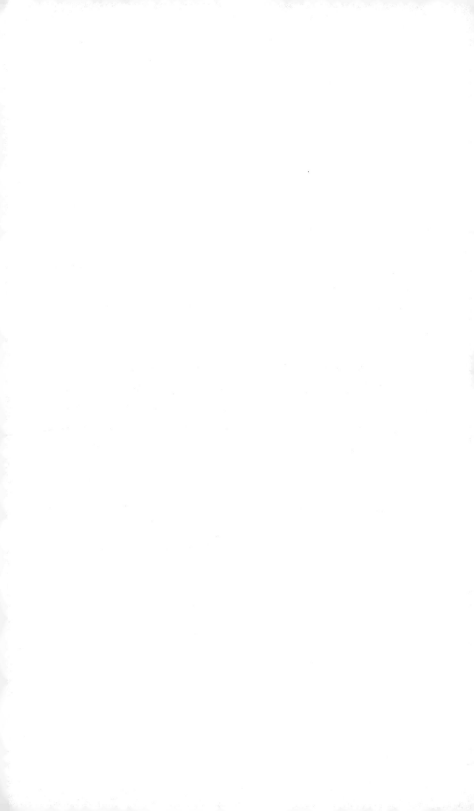

CONTENTS

ADDITIONAL RESOURCES

www.29billion.com

The above website has been created to accompany this book. It contains a range of resources and documents ready for downloading, including:

- Information on how to test blood glucose levels

- More information about customised nutrition and Metabolic Typing™

- Other resources for people who are concerned about cholesterol

- Web links to references used throughout the text

ACKNOWLEDGEMENTS

Unfortunately, nutritional science is plagued by commercial interests and propaganda from organisations that are more concerned with profit than helping people to improve their health. A degree of peer pressure also exists between experts in all fields of healthcare to conform to conventional wisdom. Over the last century a number of authors have put these concerns to one side. Where inconsistencies in a theory exist, they have refused to bow down to popular opinion and have communicated these issues without hesitation.

The information contained in this book could not have been made available if it were not for some of these authors and the incredible contributions they have made. There are far too many authors and researchers to list individually, but those who have contributed substantially to our understanding of the topics covered in this book include, but are by no means limited to: Dr Weston Price, Dr Uffe Ravnskov, Dr Roger Williams, Dr Russell Smith, Dr Malcolm Kendrick, Dr Mary Enig, Dr Charles McGee and Dr Broda Barnes.

My personal realisation of the issues discussed in this book started when I became aware of the individualised nature of nutritional requirements through Metabolic Typing™. This is a truly wonderful approach to nutrition. Over the last century a huge number of doctors and researchers have contributed to the system that is used today. In particular, William Wolcott of Healthexcel Inc has spent more than thirty years refining the system so that it produces accurate and reliable results with every person tested.

Millions of people around the world now have the opportunity to benefit from Metabolic Typing™ thanks to Bill Wolcott.

I first learnt of Metabolic Typing™ from an article written by Paul Chek (www.chekinstitute.com). This was just one of so many truly insightful articles that Paul Chek has written and I am extremely grateful to him for making a wide range of information available to all of us who have an interest in health.

If it was not for Richard Smith's shocking book *The Trouble with Medical Journals* like most, I would be unaware of the significant problems that exist within medical research. These problems affect us all.

A number of people have reviewed this book. Anyone who has attempted to write a book is aware of the critical importance of obtaining this feedback. I am indebted to Drew Leckie, Liza Zivoni, Yvonne White and Andrew Seed for their suggestions about the content. In particular, I am very grateful to Jayne Harlock at the Wellness Clinic in Chelmsford, Essex for all of her feedback on the book and generally for her encouragement and enthusiasm.

A special thank you to Nittish for accepting my lack of interest in anything but this book for at least eighteen months, and for putting up with the towers of articles and research papers in our cramped London flat. Heartfelt thanks to the Luchoomun family in Mauritius who extended extremely generous hospitality during my visit there whilst working on the book. I would also like to thank Krishna Yarlagadda generally for his insights and advice.

Last but not least, I would like to thank my loving parents for their endless support and encouragement throughout all of my endeavours.

INTRODUCTION

We are told that high cholesterol levels pose a major risk factor for developing heart disease. We are also told that the consumption of foods containing saturated fat and cholesterol increases the risk for heart disease. These statements can be summarised as: *The Cholesterol Idea.*

This book provides unequivocal evidence to show that the cholesterol idea is false and is communicated solely for the purpose of sustaining a cholesterol-lowering industry that generates around US$29 billion each year.

The reality is that cholesterol and saturated fats do not cause heart disease; these two nutrients actually protect us against heart disease and many other conditions. For the last few decades it has been convenient to blame cholesterol and saturated fat for all kinds of health problems, but when we look for the actual scientific evidence to prove that these substances are harmful, it becomes instantly clear that none exists.

The fact is that no one has ever had a heart attack simply because they have a 'high' level of cholesterol and there is no link between saturated fat in our diet and heart disease.

Heart disease is still the biggest killer in the UK and America. Efforts to reduce the incidence of heart disease have been focused on reducing saturated fat in our diet and lowering cholesterol levels. But official statistics clearly show that more people die of heart disease with low cholesterol rather than high cholesterol.

Moreover, most people who have a heart attack have an average or below average cholesterol level, not high cholesterol.

Cholesterol–lowering drugs (statins) have been portrayed as wonder drugs and are being prescribed to an increasing number of people. Millions of people who consider themselves to be healthy are being told they need to take a statin drug every day for the rest of their lives. Even worse, children as young as eight years old are now considered to be eligible for statin use according to some 'experts'.

These cholesterol-lowering drugs generate more money for the pharmaceutical industry than any other form of medication in history: reaching an unprecedented US$27.8 billion in sales in 2006. This figure is set to increase, since plans exist to screen millions more people for 'high cholesterol'.

There are a number of fundamental problems with the cholesterol idea, but these have been consistently ignored by 'experts' who support it. For example, the British Heart Foundation (BHF) tells us that cholesterol levels are too high in the UK and this represents a major cause of heart disease. This implies that cholesterol levels have risen, however data published by the BHF themselves shows that cholesterol levels have actually reduced, not increased.

The statement that cholesterol levels are high in the UK is simply not true. Even the most casual look at cholesterol levels in other countries reveals that cholesterol levels in the UK are close to the global average and low when compared with the rest of Europe.

By comparing cholesterol levels with the incidence of heart disease around the world, we can see that no correlation exists between the two. There are many countries that have a much higher average cholesterol level than the UK yet their rate of heart disease is much lower.

Other questions arise when we try to establish the cause of 'high' cholesterol. We are told that 'high' cholesterol is caused by the consumption of saturated fat. But at the same time, we are told that reducing saturated fat in our diet will not have much effect on cholesterol levels. In order to reduce cholesterol levels we are told that we have to take cholesterol-lowering drugs. This contradiction reveals the motivations behind the cholesterol idea: which is simply to make profit by turning perfectly healthy people into patients.

The business opportunities created by cholesterol phobia extend beyond the pharmaceutical industry and into the food industry. A range of new cholesterol-lowering foods have been created, such as margarines that contain plant sterols.

These plant sterols block the absorption of cholesterol and can very slightly reduce cholesterol levels. However, consumers have not been told that plant sterols also block the absorption of vital nutrients and lower levels of nutrients more than they lower cholesterol levels. Manufacturers of these products were asked by the European Commission to inform consumers about this, but they have not done so: probably because they are keen to protect a new industry for plant sterol foods that is worth more than US$1 billion.

By all accounts US$29 billion is a conservative estimate of the value of the cholesterol-lowering industry and does not include a wide range of other products created by the food industry that are capitalising on the misinformation about cholesterol.

The idea that cholesterol causes heart disease is likely to be the biggest health scam in history and a number of factors have converged to allow this to take place. These factors include: the degradation of the scientific process used in medicine, unhealthy links between medical research and pharmaceutical companies, a shift of resources in drug companies from research and development into sales and marketing, and problems with medical journals.

These factors represent a significant change in the field of medicine, where drugs are increasingly being suggested as the primary treatment option for conditions that do not require medication.

The aim of this book is to bring a number of very important health issues and associated misconceptions to the attention of the reader.

Chapter 1 provides a brief description of the types of fats in our diet, what we are told about them and why saturated fats, far from being dangerous, are vitally important for health.

Chapter 2 shows that the intake of saturated fat has been decreasing during the same time that obesity, heart disease and diabetes have been increasing. National nutritional surveys show that we are following government recommendations, but the authorities refuse to admit that these guidelines (which remain unchanged for ten years) are not working.

Chapter 3 explains how grain based foods such as bread, pasta and cereals cause obesity, diabetes, heart disease and a range of other serious health problems. Dieticians and the food industry have convinced us to double our consumption of these foods: which have significantly contributed to the decline of our health.

Chapter 4 takes a brief look at different diets around the world to show the incredible variation in the types of foods that are traditionally eaten. The importance of our genetic heritage in determining our nutritional requirements is discussed.

Chapter 5 commences with a brief description of the cholesterol idea and how it started. The false idea of 'good' and 'bad' cholesterol is also discussed.

Chapter 6 discusses the false idea that dietary cholesterol and saturated fat cause the level of cholesterol in the blood to increase.

Chapter 7 shows that the risk for developing heart disease actually increases as cholesterol levels are reduced and chapter 8 discusses the way that pharmaceutical companies and doctors are converting millions of healthy people into patients.

Chapter 9 provides a description of how the cholesterol idea has been allowed to take hold and chapter 10 asks if statins are safe.

Chapter 11 provides a basic description of how heart disease develops. The general public have been misled to believe that heart disease involves a simple process of the arteries getting 'clogged-up' with fat. In fact, we now know that the process is more akin to inflammation. A more accurate understanding of the true nature of heart disease raises even more questions about the cholesterol idea.

Chapter 12 briefly discusses some of the actual mechanisms by which high blood glucose levels cause heart disease and how this is related to diabetes.

Chapter 13 shows how clinical trials are often exaggerated and misreported to show statins as "wonder drugs". The reality is quite different from the published headlines.

Chapter 14 exposes cholesterol-lowering margarines as foods that are actually more likely to contribute to heart disease rather than prevent it. Finally, appendix A provides a brief description of what constitutes a natural whole food based diet and provides a basic food selection guide for readers.

The issues discussed in this book may be considered by many to be controversial. However, what is presented is a coherent argument against the cholesterol idea. Throughout the whole text, great care has been taken to support all statements that have been made with relevant references and source materials. These can easily be verified by the reader. The intention has been to present this important information in a way that will appeal to both the general public and those with a professional interest.

CHAPTER I

The Essential Guide to Fats

Australian Aborigines would kill a kangaroo, examine its insides for fat and if it was too lean, abandon the carcass where it lay (1-3). This practice took place for the simple reason that Aborigines fully understood the importance of fat. They had sufficient dietary wisdom to know that too much lean meat without the fat would make them sick. Eskimos accumulated the same knowledge; they discovered that if they ate too much lean deer meat without other fattier meats, they would very quickly become ill (4).

Animal fats contain various vitamins and other *activators* that are absolutely essential for good health. Some of these nutrients can also be obtained from vegetable sources, but overall animal fats provide the best source.

Nutrition is all about team work. In order for one nutrient to be absorbed and used properly, other nutrients must be present. If meat does not contain enough fat it will be lacking in certain nutrients. These nutrients provide activators for other nutrients to be assimilated. Since a full range of nutrients are required for the proper absorption of meat, the body will have to obtain any missing nutrients from its existing store. Each time very lean meat is eaten the body's store of some nutrients is further depleted. This situation can be sustained for only a short period of time until the body becomes nutritionally deficient. Eventually the body becomes weak, the immune system is compromised and disease sets in.

Dietary fats consist of a wide range of different *fatty acids*. Each of the fatty acids has a very important role to play within the body and there is still a great deal that we do not know about how each of them function. Fats are the last major essential nutrient to be examined by science and appear to be the most fascinating (5). Generally, there are three types or groups of fatty acids designated in accordance with their level of *saturation*.

Saturation refers to how closely the molecules of the fat are packed-in together. The molecules that saturated fats are made up of are more linear (or straight) and can be packed-in close together. However the molecules that unsaturated fats are made up of have kinks or bends in them, which means that they cannot be packed-in as tightly. Unsaturated fats can be *monounsaturated* or *polyunsaturated*. Polyunsaturated fats are less saturated than monounsaturated fats. This is illustrated in figure 1A.

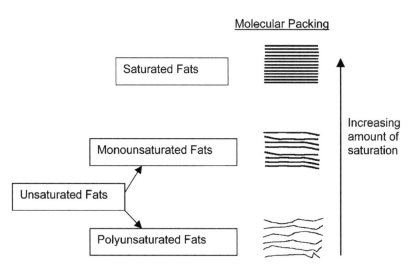

Figure 1A. Basic Illustration of Different Types of Fats

Fats are often described in terms of 'good' fats and 'bad' fats. It has become fashionable to designate saturated fats as 'bad' and unsaturated fats as 'good'. Therefore, we are advised to consume more unsaturated fats. In particular, polyunsaturated fats are promoted. However, no natural fats are intrinsically good or bad – it is the proportions that matter (6). The human body needs a wide range of different types of fats, but it may need larger quantities of some fats than others. As long as the fat has not had its molecular structure altered through processing or cooking it can be considered healthy.

Within nature, fats are provided in the form of a balance or mix of different fatty acids. No source of fat is purely saturated or purely unsaturated; rather they exist as a range of fatty acids.

Fats that are obtained from some animal sources (such as beef, lamb, chicken and pork) are generally more saturated. Hence they are called saturated fats even though they also contain unsaturated fats. In a similar way, fats from vegetable sources are called unsaturated fats because they have a predominance of unsaturated fats. Table 1A shows the basic composition of some common fats.

The degree of saturation determines how stable the fat is. For this reason saturated fats are much more stable than unsaturated fats. Polyunsaturated fats in particular are very unstable and degrade easily – meaning their molecular structure can easily be altered.

Some 'experts' tell us that we should cook with vegetable oils. However, this advice is at odds with our scientific understanding. Vegetable oils such as sunflower oil, safflower oil, and rapeseed oil are predominately polyunsaturated fats. These fats have a low melting point and are not resistant to heat.

Table 1A. Composition of Some Commonly Eaten Fats. Adapted from reference (7). Note: fats are sometimes referred to as oils. The two terms can be used interchangeably; however the term oil tends to be used when the fat is liquid at room temperature.

Type of Fat	Saturated	Monounsaturated	Polyunsaturated
Chicken Fat	31%	49%	20%
Pork Fat	40%	48%	12%
Olive Oil	13%	75%	12%
Sesame Oil	15%	42%	43%
Flax Seed Oil	9%	18%	73%

When polyunsaturated fats are heated, and when they are exposed to oxygen or sunlight, they create *free radicals*. Free radicals are unstable molecules that can attack healthy cells and lead to cancer and heart disease. Free radicals can also accelerate the aging process, cause complications with diabetes and contribute to a range of other disorders. Unfortunately, the general public are not informed that polyunsaturated fats become dangerous and should not be consumed when heated. Instead, vegetable oils are promoted ironically as healthy for the heart.

Out of all vegetable oils, only extra virgin olive oil is suitable for cooking with because it is more saturated and less refined than other vegetable oils. Butter, lard, and ghee (clarified butter) as well as coconut oil are the most saturated and hence the best fats to use for cooking. These are the fats that have been used for cooking by many generations of people, long before the food industry invented ways of making cheap oils from vegetable crops.

The molecular stability of saturated fats is put to good use within the cells of the human body. Each of the cells within the body has an outer skin or *cell membrane*. Saturated fats make up a large proportion of this membrane and provide each cell with the structure and stiffness it needs. Saturated fats also provide a valuable source of energy. In addition, they have very strong anti-viral, anti-fungal and anti-bacterial properties (8).

It is also of note that during the storage of body fat, the human body tries to protect itself from the accumulation of polyunsaturated fats by favouring fats that are more saturated. If saturated fats are unhealthy, why are they the body's preferred type of fat? Before an increased consumption of polyunsaturated fat is accepted as beneficial, an adequate explanation of this should be provided (9).

Although polyunsaturated vegetable oils are very unstable and should not generally be used for cooking, there are some polyunsaturated fats that do form an important part of the diet. Two forms of polyunsaturated fats that have received a great deal of attention are *omega 3* and *omega 6*. These are designated *essential fatty acids* (EFAs) because the body cannot make these specific fats and they must be obtained on a regular basis from our diet. Just how much omega 3 and omega 6 the human body needs is unclear, however we do know that consuming much more of one than the other is detrimental to health.

Omega 3 and omega 6 have opposing properties. Omega 3 reduces inflammation (10) and helps blood to flow more easily through vessels and arteries. This is exactly what is needed in order to prevent heart disease. However, the consumption of too much omega 3 will make it very difficult for the body to produce blood clots in the event of any damage to tissues and excessive bleeding can take place (11). This is where omega 6 comes in – it helps blood to coagulate in order to stop the bleeding at the site of an injury.

Similarly, if too much omega 6 is consumed, its properties can work against us. The coagulation can slow down the flow of blood through vessels and arteries and increase the risk for heart disease. Omega 6 can also encourage inflammation, which is another important feature of heart disease. Clearly, a balance of omega 3 and omega 6 is required so that these fats can work together to reach a compromise between their respective properties.

Most people in industrialised countries consume too much omega 6. This is because omega 6 is found in relatively large quantities in vegetable oils (such as sunflower oil) and in grain based foods such as cereals, bread and pasta. The consumption of these foods has increased drastically during the last few decades. Omega 3 however, is more difficult to obtain, the primary source being obtained from oily fish and fish oils.

An over consumption of omega 6 compared to omega 3 is associated with not only an increased risk for heart disease but also a range of other degenerative conditions (12).

CHAPTER 2

Ignorance is Bliss

The number of people dieing of heart disease is declining in most industrialised countries around the world. In the United States, between 1980 and 2000 the death rate was halved for both men and women (1). In the United Kingdom, the death rate has been declining since the 1970s (2). In England and Wales, between 1981 and 2000 there was a 62% reduction in deaths for men and a 45% reduction for women (3). This reduction in deaths is due to a combination of improvements in medical treatments and a reduction in risk factors associated with heart disease. For example, in England and Wales, most of the lives that have been saved, by far, are attributable to medical treatments (such as hospital resuscitation and medications) and people giving up smoking (3).

Although there are less people dieing of heart disease in the UK: more people are actually developing the condition. In most age groups, the number of people with heart disease is increasing. This is more apparent in older age groups (4).

The rate of diabetes is also increasing in the UK. Since 1991 the number of men with diagnosed diabetes has more than doubled and the number of women with diabetes has increased by 80% (5). It was estimated in 2007 that around 2.5 million adults in the UK have diabetes (5).

Along with heart disease and diabetes, here in the UK we also have a significant problem with obesity. This has been reported extensively in the media. The Office for National Statistics (ONS) publishes *The National Diet and Nutrition Survey*. This survey looks at the types of foods that are eaten by the population, the rate of obesity, and the incidence of other conditions. Two surveys have been completed on adults in the UK between the ages of 16 and 64 years – One survey in 1986/87 and another in 2000/01 (6).

Table 2A compares the number of people who were overweight or obese in 1986/87 with this number in 2000/01. We can see that during the fourteen year period between these two surveys an additional 21% of men and 17% of women became overweight or obese.

The three conditions mentioned above are connected. Having diabetes drastically increases the likelihood of developing heart disease. For example, women with diabetes are three to five times more likely to have heart disease (5). People with diabetes are also more likely to be overweight (7).

From a nutritional point of view, the first logical question to ask is: what have people in the UK been eating that has caused the rate

Table 2A. Increase in the Number of Overweight or Obese People in the UK between the Years 1986/87 and 2000/01. Source: The National Diet and Nutrition Survey (6).

	People Classified As Obese		People Classified As Overweight or Obese	
	MEN	WOMEN	MEN	WOMEN
1986/87 survey	8%	12%	45%	36%
2000/01 survey	25%	20%	66%	53%
	(+17%)	**(+8%)**	**(+21%)**	**(+17%)**

of heart disease, diabetes and obesity to increase? Experts tell us that too much dietary fat, and in particular, saturated fat contributes to these three conditions. According to this hypothesis, we would expect the amount of fat in the diet to have increased. However, this is not the case. In fact, the amount of fat consumed actually decreased.

The National Diet and Nutrition Survey (6) shows that between 1986/87 and 2000/01, the amount of carbohydrate in the UK diet increased and the amount of fat consumed decreased. In particular, significant reductions were seen in the consumption of saturated fat. For example, table 2B shows the percentage of total energy from carbohydrate, total fat, and saturated fat for men and women 25 to 34 years old.

The changes in the UK diet become more meaningful when we start to look at specifically which foods were eaten in larger quantities and which foods were eaten less, between the 1986/87 survey and the 2000/01 survey. The most significant changes in food consumption are summarised in Table 2C.

Table 2B. Percentage of Total Energy from Carbohydrate, Total Fat, and Saturated Fat for People Aged 25 to 34 Years in the UK Source: The National Diet and Nutrition Survey (6)

	Carbohydrate		Total Fat		Saturated Fat	
	MEN	WOMEN	MEN	WOMEN	MEN	WOMEN
1986/87	40.9%	43%	37.9%	39.4%	15.3%	16.4%
2000/01	44.6%	46.8%	33.5%	34%	12.3%	12.3%
DRV*	47%		33%		10%	

* DRV stands for 'Dietary Reference Value' and it is the estimated requirements for groups of people as specified by the British Nutrition Foundation.

Table 2C. Major Changes in the UK Diet between the 1986/87 and 2000/01 Survey. Source: The National Diet and Nutrition Survey (6)

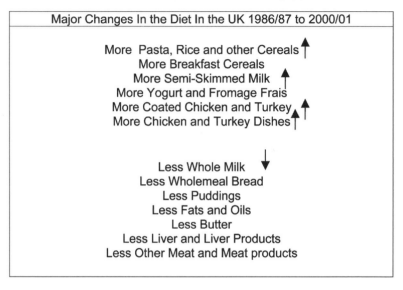

Major Changes In the Diet In the UK 1986/87 to 2000/01

More Pasta, Rice and other Cereals ↑
More Breakfast Cereals
More Semi-Skimmed Milk ↑
More Yogurt and Fromage Frais
More Coated Chicken and Turkey ↑
More Chicken and Turkey Dishes ↑

Less Whole Milk ↓
Less Wholemeal Bread
Less Puddings
Less Fats and Oils
Less Butter
Less Liver and Liver Products
Less Other Meat and Meat products

↑ Signifies a larger, more significant, increase

↓ Signifies a larger, more significant, decrease

Overall, we can see from table 2C that from 1986/87 to 2000/01 there was an obvious shift toward eating more low-fat foods. One of the most striking changes is associated with a huge increase in the amount of pasta, rice and other cereals that were eaten. In fact, the consumption of these foods went from an average of 236 grams per week in 1986/87 to 507 grams per week in 2000/01.

Overall the quantity of meat in general did not change very much but there was a huge increase in chicken and turkey based meals: which are generally lower in fat than other alternative meat products. There was also a very large shift from whole milk towards semi-skimmed milk, and a significant reduction in the amount of butter consumed.

These changes would certainly have been influenced by the national dietary recommendations. During the time between the two surveys, the main corner stone of the advice given to the public was to:

- Reduce the amount of fat in the diet
- Eat more starchy carbohydrates like pasta, rice and cereals

So, between 1986/87 and 2000/01, significant dietary changes were made in accordance with the national recommendations. Less fat (and less saturated fat), more carbohydrate (particularly more starchy carbohydrates), more semi-skimmed milk, less whole milk and less butter were consumed. However, rather than seeing a reduction in the number of people who have heart disease, diabetes, or an improvement in the obesity *figures*: we can see that the situation spiralled out of control.

It could be argued that the trends in heart disease, diabetes and obesity have been influenced by exercise and activity levels, which may have declined. To some extent this is true, and exercise / activity levels must be considered. However, the effect may not be as great as once thought. For example, data prepared for the Department of Health in England shows that men are almost as likely to be overweight or obese whether they meet the recommended activity levels or not (8).

Activity and exercise, although very important, cannot override the effects of a bad diet. If we accept that nutrition has an important role to play in the prevention of disease, we must accept that the low fat / high carbohydrate diet is not appropriate for the general population. It is clear that this diet is making things worse. Since nothing can have more of an influence on health than the food that is eaten three or more times every day, it is of paramount importance that this issue is addressed.

We might expect the authorities to ask themselves why more people become obese, develop diabetes, and suffer heart disease, when the amount of fat in the diet is reduced. However it appears that this question has been conveniently ignored.

The British Nutrition Foundation (BNF) is the main organisation within the UK that educates the general public about what constitutes healthy eating. It is stated on the BNF website (www.nutrition.org.uk) that: "Surveys such as the National Diet and Nutrition Survey series compare current intakes of nutrients with the various DRV values [Dietary Reference Values] to assess where problems exist and to assist in forming government policy" (9).

There is a very important distinction to be made here. Rather than looking at the available data from the survey and assessing the impact nutritional recommendations are having on health, the data is simply assessed in terms of how closely people are following what they have been told to do. Basically, the survey is used to check that we are following the recommendations, not if the recommendations are valid. The BNF and other organisations are not even considering that they may have got it wrong. It is not surprising then, that the obvious facts explained above have escaped attention.

The evidence for this can be seen in the current nutritional recommendations communicated by the BNF, which have not changed since the survey was completed. In fact, these recommendations have not changed for more than ten years (9). The current recommendations include:

- "Eat more starchy foods such as bread, potatoes, rice and pasta. Assuming these replace fat-containing foods, this will help to reduce the amount of fat and increase the amount of fibre in the diet. Adding fat to these foods should be avoided or kept to a minimum.
- Choosing leaner cuts of meat and lower fat versions of dairy products will help to reduce the amount of fat, particularly saturated fatty acids in the diet. Trimming fat, choosing cooking methods that do not require added fat and eating smaller portions of high fat foods can all be helpful. "(10)

This is despite the fact that there has been a definite trend for people in the UK to become more overweight, more obese, and for more people to become diabetic and suffer with heart disease: as saturated fat is reduced and more starchy carbohydrates are eaten!

During the last ten years a huge amount of nutritional research has been published. Over the last few years in particular it seems that hardly a day has passed without a nutrition related report appearing in the media. It seems strange that none of this additional knowledge requires that changes are made to the recommendations. There is a brief mention on the BNF website that the recommendations for the intake of iron, folate and selenium will be investigated (9), but in light of all the data that we now have, surely it is time for a full re-evaluation? There do not appear to be any signs of anything happening soon.

Few people have the time or the inclination to ask where our nutritional recommendations actually come from and how they are decided. We trust that the organisations responsible for this have our best interests at heart.

In the UK, nutritional requirements for particular groups of people are based on advice that was given by the Committee on Medical Aspects of Food and Nutrition Policy (COMA) in the early 1990s. Since then, COMA has been superseded by the Scientific Advisory Committee on Nutrition (SACN).

Members of SACN are required to declare any conflicts of interest. It can clearly be seen from their annual report, that many of the members of SACN have various ties with major food manufacturers, pharmaceutical companies, and even companies like weight watchers (11). There is no direct evidence that these links have influenced nutritional recommendations, but most people within the general public probably assume that the experts who set the recommendations are totally independent. The general public should be aware of these potential conflicts of interest.

It is not all that clear quite how the BNF relates to SACN, however on the BNF website it is stated that: "The British Nutrition Foundation is a registered charity. It promotes the wellbeing of society through the impartial interpretation and effective dissemination of scientifically based knowledge and advice on the relationship between diet, physical activity and health" (12).

Some people may question how "impartial" the BNF can be when they receive funding from the food industry. A list of the "Member Companies" and "Sustaining Member Companies" that support the BNF can be seen on their website (13). The BNF actually state in their company accounts that one of the objectives for the future is to increase the number of sustaining member companies and expand the membership of European based companies (14).

The BNF provides advice to consumers, schools, government departments, health professionals, industry, the scientific community and the media. Many people may feel uncomfortable about the BNF increasing its funding directly from the food industry. Although, the organisation claims to be impartial, it seems unlikely that the BNF would 'bite the hand that feeds it', and why would the member companies provide funding if they did not seek to benefit in some way?

In the next chapter and in chapter 12, we will discuss the reasons why the advice to eat more starchy foods like bread, rice and pasta is a major contributing factor to the increasing rates of heart disease, diabetes and obesity.

CHAPTER 3

More Grains: More Trouble!

Grains are a group of foods that include wheat, rice, millet, corn, spelt, rye, barley, oat, buckwheat, amaranth, quinoa, triticale and kamut. These foods are often referred to as *starchy carbohydrates* (because they contain large amounts of starch) or *complex carbohydrates* (simple sugars bonded together to form more complex structures).

The diet in the UK, America and a number of other countries contains a large proportion of grain based foods. In the UK, grains are commonly eaten in the form of bread, rice, breakfast cereals, pasta, and couscous. Grains are promoted as a healthy food. In 2005 the government listed eight recommendations for "eating well". The first recommendation in this list was "Base your meals on starchy foods" (1).

We are also told that eating grain based foods is preferable to eating foods that contain fat (2). The main reason why we are told to avoid fat is because per gram, fat contains more calories. One gram of fat contains nine calories, where as one gram of carbohydrate contains about four calories – fat is more energy dense. We are also told to avoid fat simply because there is a perception that eating fat results in the accumulation of fat on the body. Initially these arguments may seem logical: however when we look at the effects that starchy carbohydrates are known to have, the argument against fat becomes irrelevant.

First of all, we should consider the history of the consumption of grains. As we have seen from the previous chapter, there has been a large increase in the amount of grain based foods that are eaten in the UK. However, grains are a new edition to the human diet. Research shows that agriculture and grain farming have existed at most for ten to fifteen thousand years (3). This period of time is extremely short in evolutionary terms; accounting for ½ percent or less of human history. Many of us have not genetically adapted to the consumption of grains (3).

Celiac disease is an autoimmune reaction to the gluten that is contained in most grains. The inside lining of the small intestine (intestinal mucosa) becomes chronically damaged by gluten and its interaction with the immune system (3). The condition has a strong genetic connection. Our hunter-gatherer ancestors during the *Paleolithic* age did not eat grains. Their diet consisted of meat, vegetables, seeds and fruit (4). The consumption of grains that contain gluten started during the *Neolithic* period in Turkey, Iran, Iraq, Israel / Palestine, Syria, and Lebanon (4). Later spreading to other parts of the world.

At the time when grains were first eaten, celiac disease may not have been a huge problem. The degree of damage to the intestinal wall is related to the amount and timing of gluten ingestion. In the past, infants may have had prolonged breast feeding, which would have meant that the consumption of gluten would have started later in life (4). This and other factors meant that gluten consumption may have followed a different pattern than that of today: where the consumption of gluten grains has increased drastically, and is still increasing.

The second point to consider is that although carbohydrates like grains contain less calories per gram, if we eat too much of them, they are in any case, converted into fat within the body and stored as excess body fat. Grain based foods do not provide the same level of satiety as foods containing protein and fat. Studies have found that people on a high protein and fat diet spontaneously reduce their calorie intake (5). Some experts have suggested that the reduced calorie intake is due to a restricted diet but there is no evidence of this at all. On the contrary, a high protein and fat diet includes a full array of meats, poultry, seafood, beans, pulses, eggs, cheese, vegetables, and some fruits. Where as, a grain based low-fat diet can in some cases be quite bland.

Television advertisements (particularly for breakfast cereals) along with many dieticians, like to promote complex carbohydrates like grains as a 'slow-releasing' form of energy. Describing grains, even whole grains (which are unrefined grains) as a slow-releasing form of energy is deceptive and simply inaccurate. Since grains are not slow-releasing at all.

The term slow-releasing refers to the effect that foods have on blood sugar levels after they are eaten. When carbohydrates are eaten they enter the blood stream as glucose (sugar) and cause blood glucose levels to increase. Some carbohydrates will cause blood glucose to rise more quickly than others.

Carbohydrates are often given a *glycemic index* or *GI value*, which relates to their effect on blood glucose – generally, the higher the GI value of a food, the more it will raise blood glucose levels.

Some experts prefer to use *glycemic load* which takes into account the amount of carbohydrate in a typical serving size of the food as well as its inherent GI value. Again, the higher the glycemic load, the more the food will raise blood glucose levels. Table 3A lists the GI and glycemic load values for some commonly eaten foods.

It can be seen from table 3A, that the glycemic load provides a more practical estimation of the effects a food will have on blood glucose levels. For example, spaghetti and green peas both have a similar GI value, however, in reality: spaghetti may cause blood glucose levels to rise much more than green peas. This is because spaghetti contains more carbohydrate than green peas. In addition, spaghetti tends to be eaten in larger quantities than green peas. Green peas are usually eaten in small quantities to accompany a meal, where as spaghetti often constitutes the main part of the meal. For these reasons the glycemic load of spaghetti is much higher than that of green peas. In practical terms this is more useful to know than just the GI value.

The degree any given carbohydrate will raise blood glucose levels varies considerably between different people. This is illustrated

Table 3A. The Glycemic Index and Glycemic Load of Some Commonly Eaten Foods

Food	Glycemic Index	Glycemic Load (Serving Size)
French Baguette	95	15 (30 grams)
Cornflakes™	77	21 (30 grams)
Bran Flakes™	50	10 (30 grams)
White Bread	70	10 (30 grams)
Wholemeal Bread	69	8 (30 grams)
Spaghetti	44	20 (180 grams)
Green Peas	48	3 (80 grams)
Apple	39	6 (120 grams)
Butter Beans	28	5 (150 grams)
Peanuts	14	1 (50 grams)
Carrot, raw	16	1 (80 grams)

in figure 3A, which compares the blood glucose levels of sixteen different people after consuming foods that are low in their GI value and foods that have a high GI value. It can be seen that in one person the high GI diet doubled their level of blood glucose, but in other people there was no significant difference, and in a small number of cases it was actually the low GI diet that increased blood glucose more.

It is important to note that the low GI and high GI diets used in the study illustrated in figure 3A only differed slightly. The low GI diet included foods such as porridge and pasta, where as the high GI diet included processed cereals and potatoes. The low GI diet was only 15% lower in GI value than the high GI diet. There were no differences in the amount of protein, fat and carbohydrate

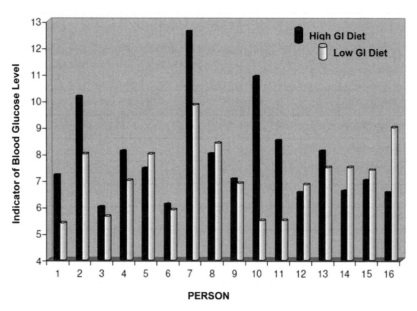

Figure 3A. The Effect of a High GI and Low GI Diet on Blood Glucose in Sixteen People. Blood Glucose is measured by Glycosylated Hemoglobin Percentage. Adapted from reference (6).

between the two diets. This shows that some reduction in blood glucose can often be achieved by substituting one type of carbohydrate for another type.

This is the idea behind the promotion of grain based foods as slow-releasing forms of energy. We are led to believe that grains have a low glycemic load when compared with other foods, but this is simply not true. For a start, there are many alternative carbohydrates (mainly vegetables) that have a lower glycemic load, and will not increase blood glucose levels as much as grains do. More significantly however is the fact that protein and fat have much less effect on blood glucose levels than any carbohydrates.

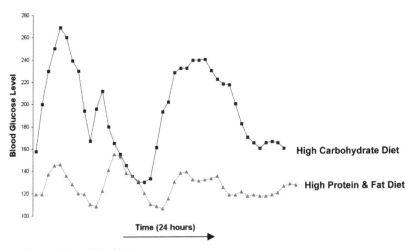

Composition of the Diets

	High Carbohydrate Diet	High Protein & Fat Diet
Carbohydrate	55%	20%
Protein	15%	30%
Fat	30%	50%

Figure 3B. The Effects of a High Carbohydrate and a High Protein and Fat Diet on Blood Glucose Levels during a 24 Hour Period. Adapted from reference (7).

When we look at the effect that an overall meal will have on blood glucose levels it is essential to consider the amount of protein, fat and carbohydrate that is eaten, not just the type of carbohydrate. Since meals that contain more protein and fat (and by definition less carbohydrate) will have much less effect on blood glucose levels. This is illustrated in figure 3B.

It can be seen from figure 3B that not only does a high carbohydrate diet result in much higher blood glucose levels than a high protein and fat diet, but it also causes marked fluctuations in blood glucose levels.

Some readers will be familiar with the *GI Diet*, which is a nutrition program based on selecting carbohydrates that have a lower GI value. A number of diet books and cook books have been written for the GI Diet, one of the more popular ones has been written by Rick Gallop (8). In some ways the GI Diet is a step in the right direction, however, there are serious limitations with it. The most significant problem is that the GI Diet promotes a low-fat diet that is very high in carbohydrate. Choosing carbohydrates that have a lower GI value can help to reduce blood glucose levels but for many people, the only way to gain control over their blood glucose levels is to reduce their overall carbohydrate intake and consume more protein and fat. Figure 3C provides an overall representation of the effects that different food groups have on blood glucose levels. Substituting one carbohydrate based food for another type of carbohydrate that has a lower GI is helpful, but increasing the intake of protein and fat based foods has much more of a desirable effect.

Promoters of the GI Diet claim that dietary fat leads to the accumulation of body fat: however, as we shall see in the next section, it is actually a diet that is too high in carbohydrate content that is much more likely to lead to weight gain.

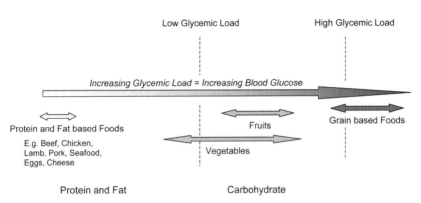

Figure 3C. Overall Representation of the Effects Different Food Groups Have on Blood Glucose Levels.

Different people will react very differently to the same amount of carbohydrate in a meal. This is due to the large variation in the way that foods are converted into energy between different people. Each person has their own unique metabolic individuality. This subject is discussed in more detail in the next chapter. The main point to be made here is that for many people, increasing the amount of grain based foods in a meal will drastically increase the glycemic load of that meal, causing blood glucose levels to increase - especially if grains are being added instead of foods containing fat – as is recommended by dieticians. This has a number of very serious and potentially dangerous implications.

How Grains Make Us Fat

All farmers know that if you feed cattle on grains they get fat more quickly. This is one of the main reasons why most beef that is bought in the supermarket is from cattle that have been fed on grains. Cows are designed to eat grass but when their entire diet is made up of grains (like wheat and corn) the animals often become sick and the quality of the fats and protein from their meat declines (9). Animals fed on grains have from one- third to three times more fat on them than animals fed on grass (10). Not that fat is bad per se, but this illustrates the fact that grains make animals fatter quicker. The problem is that grains make humans fat as well.

The amount of glucose in the blood stream has to be regulated as an absolute priority. If the level drops below 40 mg/dl (milligrams per decilitre) or 2.2 mmol/l (millimoles per litre), coma, seizure, or death can occur. Levels exceeding about 180 mg/dl or 10mmol/l are associated with heart disease and kidney failure (11). Therefore the body has a regulatory system that aims to keep blood glucose levels under control. This regulatory system is provided by two hormones, namely: *insulin* and *glucagon*.

The main role of insulin is to enable the body to use glucose. Carbohydrates are broken down in the stomach and intestines and enter the blood stream as glucose. This triggers the release of insulin from the pancreas. Insulin transports glucose to cells where it can be used for immediate use as energy. Insulin is also involved in converting excess glucose into stored body fat and helps glucose to be stored in the liver for future use.

Glucagon is responsible for the opposite actions of insulin – it releases glucose from the liver and releases fat from storage to be used for energy.

Under normal circumstances these two opposing hormones keep blood glucose levels under control. However if too much carbohydrate is eaten, or a meal is consumed that has a high gylcemic load, the regulatory mechanism becomes imbalanced. The release of insulin is proportional to the increase in the blood glucose level. Therefore, a high blood glucose level results in a large amount of insulin being released. A high level of insulin actually suppresses the release of glucagon. This state of high insulin and low glucagon stimulates the storage of glucose in the liver and promotes the accumulation of more body fat. It also means that existing body fat cannot be broken down (11).

Eventually the release of glucose into the blood stream (from the food that has been consumed) starts to slow down, however the high level of insulin in the blood persists. This means that the blood glucose level now drops to a low level. This condition is known as *hypoglycaemia*. This state of hypoglycaemia triggers a feeling of hunger and another dose of carbohydrate or high glycemic index food is usually eaten to boost the blood glucose level – and the cycle continues again.

Eating too much carbohydrate or meals with a high glycemic load can easily create continuous cycles of high blood glucose followed by hypoglycaemia that continue throughout the whole day. Effectively the person becomes overly reliant on glucose for energy and is unable to 'burn' body fat. The presence of large amounts of insulin in the blood effectively 'switches off' the ability to use stored body fat. This combined with the additional hunger created by the periods of hypoglycaemia (leading to more food being eaten) results in weight gain.

A study published in the *New England Journal of Medicine* followed 85,941 women between the ages of 34 and 59 years (12). It was found that between 1980 and 1990, the glycemic load of the diet they consumed had increased by 22%. During the same time period the number of women who were overweight increased 38%.

With all of this in mind, it is no surprise that when a high carbohydrate diet is compared with a low carbohydrate diet, people who follow the low carbohydrate diet, that includes larger amounts of protein and fat, usually loose more weight. This is what has been found in at least seven published trials (13-19). For example, one of these studies found that people on the low carbohydrate diet lost on average 5.8Kg, where as the people on the low-fat / high carbohydrate diet lost an average of 1.9Kg (18).

This certainly does not mean that a low carbohydrate / high protein and fat diet is appropriate for everyone. As stated earlier, how each of us reacts to a high carbohydrate meal is determined by our metabolic individuality. Some people are suited to a high carbohydrate diet, where as others are suited to a low carbohydrate diet. Our nutritional requirements are dictated to a large extent by our genetic heritage. Problems occur when we eat too many carbohydrates for our own individual metabolic machinery to cope with.

Diabetes

There are two kinds of diabetes: *type 1* and *type 2*. Type 1 diabetes usually appears very early on in life and is related to the inability of the pancreas to make insulin. Type 1 diabetes is often called *insulin-dependent diabetes* because people with the condition have to take daily injections of insulin. Type 2 diabetes usually develops in later life and is much more common than Type 1. Up to ninety percent of people with diagnosed diabetes have the type 2 variety (20). People with type 2 diabetes can be deficient in the amount of insulin that is produced by the pancreas, but they are not dependent on insulin injections. The way that the body uses insulin can also be impaired in type 2 diabetes.

There are also some people who are in a situation known as being *prediabetic*: this means that the effects of insulin are impaired but not to the degree that is associated with a diagnosis of diabetes.

As we have seen, insulin is needed to lower blood glucose levels. Therefore diabetes of all kinds is characterised by an inability to lower blood glucose levels after the consumption of carbohydrate. The primary goal in the management of diabetes is to gain control over the amount of glucose in the blood. It is absurd then, that most diabetics are told to eat a low fat, high carbohydrate diet – the very diet that will raise their blood glucose levels!

Diabetics may be told to avoid eating fat because of a fear that dietary fat will make them gain weight. However, as we have seen in the section above, this is a misconception and in fact, too much carbohydrate in the diet is more likely to result in gaining weight. It is no surprise that most people who have diabetes are also overweight - those people who are susceptible to having high blood glucose levels while following a diet that is high in carbohydrate will be at risk for both gaining weight and developing diabetes.

When we continue to consume too much carbohydrate, the body has to keep making more insulin in an attempt to reduce blood glucose levels. This results in a high level of insulin in the blood stream. The cells of the body respond to this high level of insulin in the blood by decreasing the number of *insulin receptors* on their membranes (21). Insulin receptors are like tiny docking devices or landing sites for insulin. They are positioned on the outer layer of cells. When insulin reaches a docking device (receptor) it triggers the sequence of biochemical processes that enable glucose to be used by the cell.

The reduction in the number of insulin receptors effectively means that the cells are resistant to insulin. This resistance occurs because insulin cannot act upon the cells without its receptors being available. Medically, this state is known as *insulin resistance.*

Insulin resistance prevents the lowering of blood glucose levels. But the blood glucose level may still be too high, so the pancreas has to release even more insulin into the blood stream. The cells will respond by becoming more insulin resistant and a vicious circle of events develops. This cycle may continue for a number of days, weeks or even years. This is illustrated in figure 3D.

The continued production of high levels of insulin also prevents the release of stored body fat and results in weight gain. Increased body fat may lead to more insulin resistance: making the situation even worse.

Insulin is produced by cells in the pancreas called *beta cells.* Several studies have demonstrated that the increased demand for insulin and high levels of insulin in the blood can directly impact upon the function of beta cells (11). High blood glucose can also damage beta cells.

The excess glucose in the blood is converted into a type of fat called a *triglyceride.* Too many triglycerides in the blood can also damage beta cells (11). Eventually the beta cells can become exhausted and unable to produce enough insulin, which further impairs the body's ability to lower blood glucose levels – leading to a diagnosis of diabetes.

Other effects that a high carbohydrate diet can have on diabetes are discussed in chapter 12.

Glycohemoglobin, also known as *glycosylated haemoglobin,* is a measure of the long term control of diabetes. A normal level of

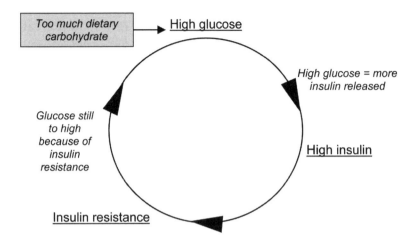

Figure 3D. The Vicious Circle of Events Leading to Diabetes

glycohemoglobin is less than 7%, and levels above 9% show poor control of diabetes. A study published in the journal *Diabetes* found that a high carbohydrate diet maintained existing levels of glycohemoglobin in people with type 2 diabetes, but a high protein and fat diet significantly reduced glycohemoglobin (7). By following the high protein and fat diet, a reduction was seen by the end of the first week, and after five weeks a reduction of 22% in glycohemoglobin was achieved (from 9.8% to 7.6%).

Grains and Heart Disease

A high level of triglycerides in the blood can not only contribute to diabetes but it can also increase the risk for heart disease. High triglyceride levels have been associated with heart disease for many years. Some researchers hold the opinion that high triglyceride levels directly increase the risk for heart disease, independently of other risk factors. Other experts have focussed on the fact that a high level of triglycerides results in a greater number of *small dense LDL (low density lipoprotein) particles* that are more likely to become oxidised. The dangers associated with small dense LDLs are discussed in chapter 12.

Both the British Heart Foundation and Heart UK advise people to lower their triglyceride levels in order to reduce the risk for heart disease (22, 23). However, both organisations also state that eating too much fat is the cause of having high triglycerides. Simply because a triglyceride is a type of fat, it is suggested that dietary fat will cause high blood levels of triglycerides. In fact, high levels of triglycerides are actually caused by having an excess of carbohydrates in the diet; not fat. This is because the excess glucose in the blood stream (resulting from the consumption of too much carbohydrate) has to be converted into triglycerides, which are then stored in the body's fat cells.

It is important to state that this mechanism of converting excess blood glucose into triglycerides is a simple fact of biology, and is not disputed. It is also important to realise that there are at least twelve published scientific studies to show that a high carbohydrate diet results in considerably higher levels of triglycerides and a high protein and fat diet actually reduces triglyceride levels (13-15, 17-19, 24-29). High protein and fat diets produce fewer triglycerides in the blood stream mainly because they do not cause the same rapid fluctuations in blood glucose levels that a high carbohydrate diet does for a lot of people.

In addition to the adverse effects on triglyceride levels, high blood glucose directly increases the risk for heart disease by damaging the arteries that supply blood to the heart. Some of the mechanisms involved in this process are discussed in chapter 12.

Scientific Research Proves the Ill Effects of High Glucose

A large number of studies have established blood glucose levels as an independent risk factor for cardiovascular disease (any problem with the heart or blood vessels) and death from any cause. Of particular significance is the fact that high blood glucose increases these risks in people who do not have diabetes as well as those who do have diabetes (30-41).

Researchers measured the blood glucose levels of 1860 Swedish men and followed their health history for more than 17 years. It was found that an increase in blood glucose correlated with an increased risk for having a heart attack (30).

A study published in the journal *Diabetes Care* included a national sample of 3092 American adults. After the 16 year follow up period, people with high blood glucose had a two fold increased risk of dieing. High blood glucose increased the death rate for all causes and cardiovascular causes (31).

Another study included 582 people who were at risk for type 2 diabetes and found that blood glucose was strongly associated with signs of heart disease (33).

Researchers from Harvard Medical School conducted an investigation on 75,521 women who did not have diabetes. It was found that a higher glycemic load and an increase in carbohydrate intake were associated with an increase in the rate of heart disease. It was also found that reducing saturated fat intake actually increased the risk for heart disease. Women in the high carbohydrate group had 186 cases of heart disease; where as those with the lowest carbohydrate intake had 139 cases (35).

Another investigation established that high blood glucose levels, but still lower than the threshold for a diagnosis of diabetes, are associated with a 27% greater risk for cardiovascular disease (36).

A study published in the *Lancet* in 2006 collated data on blood glucose and cardiovascular disease from 52 countries. In addition to the 959,000 deaths directly assigned to diabetes, 1,490,000 deaths from heart disease, and 709,000 deaths from stroke, were attributable to high blood glucose. The total number of deaths related to higher than optimum blood glucose was comparable to the number of deaths from smoking (37).

Overall there is an almost linear progression in the risk for heart

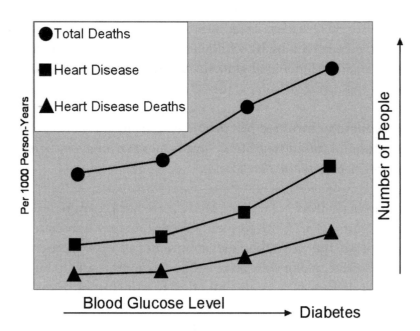

Figure 3E. The Effects of Increasing Blood Glucose Levels on Heart Disease, Heart Disease Death Rate and Total Death Rate from All Causes. Source: Reference (39)

disease, cardiovascular disease and death as blood glucose levels increase (39, 40). This is illustrated in figure 3E.

From the scientific evidence we have available to us, it is very clear that increasing the glycemic load of the diet, for many people, will significantly increase the risk for disease and death. Increasing the consumption of grain based foods leads to an excess of carbohydrate in the diet and directly increases the glycemic load. Thus, existing dietary recommendations can only have the effect of placing more people at risk.

It is understandable that we make the mistake of thinking that simply eating dietary fat will lead to weight gain and heart disease. After all, at first appearance this seems logical. However, we now have an abundance of scientific knowledge and epidemiological data to show that dietary fat is not the villain. Our ability to reduce the incidence of diabetes, obesity and heart disease depends on our ability to break free from the misplaced prejudice against dietary fat.

Grains are Nutritionally Inferior

Aside from all of the problems discussed above, grains are also one of the most nutritionally inferior foods we have available to us. For example, if we look at the vitamin content of foods, it is clear that meat, poultry and fish provide the best source for most of the vitamins – being the best source for vitamin A, D, B1, B2, B3, B6, B12, Pantothenic Acid, vitamin K2 and Biotin. The only three vitamins that animal proteins and fats do not provide the best source for are vitamin C, K, and Folic Acid – these three have to come from vegetables and fruit (42). In fact, one of the best sources of vitamin C is the adrenal glands of animals. This part of the animal was revered by our ancestors for its nutritional qualities, but unfortunately, this knowledge has been forgotten in the industrialised world: placing a greater dependency on vegetables and fruit for vitamin C.

Table 3B lists the best dietary sources for each of the vitamins. It can be seen that grains hardly feature at all in this list.

Tables detailing the best dietary source for a particular vitamin can vary. Depending on the serving size that is used for comparison, along with other factors, some references specify a slightly different list of foods. However, it is well established that proteins from animal sources provide the best source of nearly all the vitamins.

Many of these vitamins are essential for proper functioning of the heart and blood vessels. The best way to ensure adequate intake of these is to consume sufficient quantities of good quality meats, poultry, fish and vegetables. Why would anyone wish to fill their diet with foods, such as grains, that are low in essential nutrients? The food industry and many dieticians would have us believe that grains are needed to provide energy for the body. If this is the case, then how did we manage to survive for the other 99.5% of human history without grains in our diet?

Whole Grains verses Refined Grains

Grains come in *kernels* that consist of three parts: the *germ*, *endosperm*, and the *bran*. The germ and endosperm are contained inside the bran. These are commonly known as *whole grains* and they are used to make foods such as wholemeal bread and whole wheat pasta. Whole grain foods are often promoted as healthy

Table 3B. Foods Providing the Best Source for Various Vitamins

Nutrient	Best Sources
Vitamin B1	Beef kidney, pork, eggs
Vitamin B2	Organ meats, beef, pork, lamp, milk, broccoli, eggs, poultry, fish
Vitamin B3	Beef, chicken, pork, and lamp, liver, swordfish, tuna, halibut
Vitamin B5 Pantothenic Acid	Beef, pork, lamb, chicken liver, eggs, herring, peanuts, bran
Vitamin B6	Liver of beef, chicken, pork, herring, mackerel, salmon, eggs, walnuts
Vitamin B12	Liver and kidney, lamb, poultry, pork, beef. egg yoke, crab, salmon, sardines, herring, oysters
Biotin	Pork liver, egg yoke
Vitamin A	Beef liver, broccoli, cantaloupe, parsley, turnips, egg yoke, milk, cheese, butter, fish
Vitamin D	Cod liver oil, egg yoke, lard, shrimp, tuna
Folic Acid	Green leafy vegetables, liver, asparagus
Vitamin C	Green peppers, parsley, broccoli, brussels sprouts, strawberries, citrus fruits
Vitamin E	Wheat germ, sunflower seeds, asparagus, broccoli, cabbage, other green leafy vegetables, whole grains
Vitamin K	Cabbage, kale, spinach, cauliflower, tomatoes, peas, carrots, liver
Vitamin K2	Organ meats, full-fat cheese, butter, cream, egg yoke. The probiotic (friendly) bacteria in the gut also produce this vitamin

foods, however these claims are made mostly in relation to their benefits over sugary foods and refined gain products.

Refined grains are processed to have their bran and germ removed. These grains are made into products such as white bread, white flour, white rice, cakes and pastries. The process of refining increases the self life of these products but also drastically reduces their nutritional content. For example, if we look at mineral content, white flour contains only 13% of the chromium, 9% of the manganese, 19% of the iron, 30% of the cobalt, 10-30% of the copper, 17% of the zinc, 50% of the molybdenum, and 17% of the magnesium found in wholewheat (43). Vitamin content is reduced in a similar way. Refined grain products also have a higher glycemic index. For example, French baguette (made of white flour) and wholemeal bread have a glycemic index of 95 and 69 respectively.

Some refined grain products are enriched or fortified with vitamins in an attempt to put back some of the lost nutrients. Unfortunately, the bioavailability of these added nutrients is extremely low because synthetic forms are often used that the body cannot absorb very well. Judith DeCava in her book *The Real Truth about Vitamins and Anti-Oxidants* provides a thorough evaluation of the problems associated with using synthetic forms of vitamins (44).

Foods that are made from refined grains are *anti-nutrients*. This means that they actually take more out of the body than they provide the body with. In order for foods to be digested and synthesised within the cells of the body, a whole range of vitamins, minerals, and enzymes are needed. Human metabolism involves a complex step by step conversion of raw materials into different biochemical substances. At each stage in the process, specific nutrients are required.

For example, carbohydrates require *B vitamins* in order for them to be synthesised properly. If these nutrients are not provided by the foods that have been eaten in a meal, then they have to be obtained from the body's existing store of nutrients. As we have seen, refined grains are not accompanied by nutrients in the quantities that nature intended them to contain, so when we eat them regularly, we eventually become deficient in vital nutrients.

Whole grain foods are healthier than the refined variety, but compared with refined grain products almost any food stuff will seem healthy. Whole grains may have more nutrients and less adverse effects on blood glucose levels than refined grains, but they are still far inferior to the full range of meats, poultry, fish, vegetables and fruit that the human race has thrived on for hundreds of thousands of years.

The food industry promotes some whole grain foods as 'healthy for the heart'. This is another way of misleading the consumer. Whole grains are better for the heart than refined grains but, as we have seen, all grains have the potential to cause high blood glucose levels and increase the risk for obesity, diabetes and heart disease.

Whole Grains Block the Absorption of Minerals

Overall, whole grains are healthier than refined grains, but another fact that the manufacturers of whole grain foods do not tell consumers is that whole grains block the absorption of minerals in the digestive system. The minerals that are blocked include: calcium, magnesium, iron, copper and zinc. Regular consumption of whole grains can lead to deficiencies in these nutrients over time. This is due to substances that are contained in the bran of grains, such as *phytic acid* and *fibre* (45).

It has been known for decades that bran inhibits the absorption of minerals. For example, a study was published in the *Lancet* in 1942 showing that less iron was absorbed when bread with a high bran content was consumed (46). Other studies have shown that wholemeal bread reduces the level of zinc in the blood stream (47).

Swedish researchers published a study in the *American Journal of Clinical Nutrition* in 1987 showing that bran can reduce iron absorption by more than 39%. The researchers concluded "There is no doubt that wheat bran inhibits the absorption of iron in man" (48).

Many 'experts' indiscriminately recommend increasing the fibre content of the diet. The fibre content of whole grains is promoted as a selling feature during advertisements for breakfast cereals, and fibre is often described as being protective against a wide range of diseases. Although some people benefit from fibre in the diet, for others, fibre can actually cause problems for the digestive system (42). Fibre is also known to inhibit the absorption of minerals. It binds with minerals and prevents them from being absorbed (47). One study found that the zinc contained in beef is four times more easily absorbed by the human body than the zinc contained in a high fibre bran flake breakfast cereal (45). This was due to fibre, phytic acid and potentially other zinc inhibitors found in bran.

For many people the ill effects of these mineral blockers in bran will not lead to significant problems as long as grains feature as a small part of the overall diet. However, if grain consumption continues to increase (as recommended by many dieticians) we can only expect an increase in mineral deficiencies.

Traditionally, grains were soaked or fermented before they were prepared for eating. These processes neutralise many of the mineral blockers contained in grains, and in effect, predigest grains so that their nutrients become more available (49). Of course, modern processing methods do not include soaking or fermenting stages since it is very time consuming. However, specially prepared *sprouted grain* breads and *sourdough breads* are sometimes available, which have been processed in a way to remove many of their mineral blockers and are superior in quality to other breads.

Brain Chemicals

Substituting foods that contain fat for grain based foods (as recommended by dieticians) will reduce the amount of protein from meat, poultry and fish in the diet. This may lead to a deficiency in vitally important *neurotransmitters*.

When the brain sends a signal to the rest of the body, it is communicated via chemical messengers that actually jump across from one nerve cell to another. These chemical messengers or brain chemicals are called neurotransmitters. The brain uses neurotransmitters to tell the heart to beat, the lungs to breathe, and the stomach to digest food.

Deficiencies in neurotransmitters can cause a wide range of symptoms. For example, serotonin is one of the neurotransmitters and low levels of serotonin may be linked with obesity, carbohydrate cravings and insomnia (50, 51).

Neurotransmitters are actually made from proteins: particularly animal proteins such as meat, poultry and fish. When the body is overly stressed, it can use up these neurotransmitters more quickly and place greater demands for the proteins that are needed as raw materials to make them. Therefore, a diet that is low in animal protein foods can lead to a deficiency in neurotransmitters.

Final Note on Grains

In the above discussion, all grains have been grouped together, but there are differences between them. Some grains are worse than others in terms of their glycemic effects, nutrient content, protein content and phytic acid content. Also, the effects of a particular grain or grain based food on an individual person are determined by a number of factors relating to genetic heritage and differences in metabolism. Some people will be able to tolerate some types of grains but not other types. The amount of grains that can be eaten by an individual person is also determined by their individual metabolism.

The main aim of this chapter is to clearly demonstrate that the recommendation to eat more grains will, for most people, significantly increase the risk for obesity, diabetes and heart disease. Much of this increased risk is related to the consequential increase in carbohydrate consumption, but other problems relate to the specific effects that grains have on the body: which can compound these risks.

The suggestion here is not that everyone should immediately stop eating all grains. These foods can form part of the diet for some people, but they certainly should not form the major part of the diet for anyone!

CHAPTER 4

Different People: Different Diets

Reports about diet and nutrition are fraught with contradiction. Yesterday's 'superfood' becomes today's cancer causing food. If we ask for advice about nutrition from three different sources, we will probably get three different answers. It is no wonder that some people have given-up and do not know where to turn for advice about healthy eating.

A multi-billion pound diet industry has emerged that includes an exhaustive range of fad diets. One of the main differences between each of these diets concerns the proportions of carbohydrate, protein and fat that is recommended. Some experts recommend a low carbohydrate/high protein and fat approach, where as others advocate a high carbohydrate/low protein and fat program. The recommendations between different diets can be poles apart yet each program has numerous success stories in support of it. How can completely opposite approaches achieve the same results?

When the authorities establish nutritional recommendations for a whole nation, they attempt to provide a simple 'one size fits all' set of guidelines. This certainly makes their job easier but unfortunately it bears no relation to the realities of nutritional science. If we look around the world we can see that different cultures have historically eaten very different kinds of foods. Genetically people adapted to the range of foods that were available to them in their immediate environment. Nutritional wisdom was passed down from one generation to the next and each successive generation remained healthy.

During the 1920s and 1930s a dentist by the name of Dr Weston Price travelled around the world to study the foods eaten by traditional cultures. His work is summarised in a classic book titled *Nutrition and Physical Degeneration* (1). This book is very highly recommended to anyone who has an interest in health. Dr. Price studied a great variety of different cultures from North American Indians to Australian Aborigines and New Zealand Maori.

Within each of the cultures he studied, Dr Price found that people stayed healthy as long as they stick to their traditional diets – the foods that were eaten by their ancestors. However, whenever a group of people tried to follow a different diet, and in particular, consumed processed 'modern' foods, they became affected by the degenerative conditions that plague the industrialised world.

Our metabolisms evolve over tens of thousands of years. Modern technology has allowed people to migrate across vast distances but during this time our metabolic makeup has not changed significantly. Here in the UK, as with many other countries around the world, we have a real 'melting pot' of cultures and genetic heritage. This has resulted in a wide range of different nutritional requirements. Some people may be suited to the general high carbohydrate/low fat diet that is recommended to everyone. However, many other people will not be suited to this and they may need much more protein and fat than carbohydrate in order to achieve optimum health.

Over the last few decades experts have been trying to find the villain in our food. Some say it is carbohydrate, and others blame fat. As we have already seen, dietary saturated fat and cholesterol have bore the brunt of this narrow minded approach. However, an assessment of nutrition from a global perspective reveals a number of case studies that may help us to learn more about the link between what we eat and our health. The purpose of this chapter is to discuss a few of these examples that demonstrate the need for an individualised approach to nutrition.

Alaskan Eskimos

In the early 1920s Dr Victor Levine from the Creighton School of Medicine planned a trip to Alaska to study the health of native Eskimos. In a *New York Times* article he was quoted as saying: "The Eskimos seem to be more capable of resisting disease and hardships than those of more southern climates. Yet they defy all the known laws of nutrition. They eat large amounts of protein and fats, but are short on other vital elements without which we in this part of the world could not live at all for any length of time" (2).

Indeed, the native Eskimo at this time was highly admired for having excellent health. Dr Western Price also commented on the health of the native Eskimo, by stating that it was amongst the best that he had encountered on his travels, and that he was "deeply concerned to know the formula of his [the Eskimos'] nutrition in order that we may learn from it" (1).

Another researcher: Dr Cleave, a surgeon captain in the Royal Navy, was interested in the low rate of heart disease in Eskimo communities. Dr Cleave observed that the Eskimo followed a highly carnivorous diet, being abundant in meat and fat, yet there was an absence of heart disease (3).

Dr Cleave studied many traditional cultures around the world.

He documented the importance of wholesome natural foods and an evolutionary approach to nutrition. In particular, he was concerned with the effect of consuming refined carbohydrates such as white flour. These investigations led to the discovery of what Cleave referred to as the *incubation period* for degenerative disease. This is related to the amount of time it takes for signs of disease to become apparent within a community, after people start consuming refined carbohydrates. Cleave generally found that this incubation period was 20 years for diabetes and 30 years for heart disease.

Back in 1974, when Dr Cleave published his book summarising his research (3), he had already begun to understand the mechanism by which high blood glucose (sugar) levels damage the arteries and cause heart disease. He also commented on the absurdity of the idea that saturated fat causes heart disease – stating that this idea has no logical foundation from an evolutionary point of view.

The findings of Dr Levine, Dr Price, Dr Cleave and many others, have since been confirmed by the increasing rates of disease in all countries that increasingly adopt refined foods and abandon traditional foods. Of the many examples of this, the story of the Eskimo is amongst the most striking. Since when native Eskimos abandon their traditional eating patterns and follow a western diet their rate of diabetes and heart disease increases drastically.

Native Eskimos in America now have a higher rate of disease than the general population. Having once been studied for their incredibly low rates of diabetes and heart disease, Eskimos who eat western foods suddenly become at high risk for these diseases. For example, native Eskimos are now 2.3 times more likely to have diabetes, 1.6 times more likely to be obese, and 1.2 times more likely to have heart disease than their white American counterparts (4).

The decline in the health of native Eskimos has been more rapid than what has been seen in most other cultures. But this was predicted by Dr Price decades ago and it is exactly what would be expected when we look at nutrition from an evolutionary point of view. As stated above, the traditional diet followed by Eskimos consisted mostly of protein and fat based foods. These foods included large quantities of dried salmon (as each piece of fish was broken off it was dipped in seal oil), fish eggs, whale skin and the organs of sea animals. Other foods included caribou, nuts, kelp, and cranberries (1).

Native Eskimos from Alaska are given the same nutritional guidelines as the rest of the American public. They are advised to eat more fruits and vegetables (up to nine servings a day), eat whole grains, cut down on fatty foods and limit the amount of fat in their diet (5, 6)

Dieticians and other 'experts' focus on reducing the fat content of the diet, but surely attention should be given to the dissimilarities between the traditional Eskimo diet and the one which is now being advised. Traditionally, the Eskimo would simply not have any grain based foods available to them. Neither would they have access to the majority of fruits and vegetables that are found in warmer climates. Their metabolisms have evolved to thrive on protein and fat based foods – the foods that were available to them. Otherwise these people would not have survived.

It is curious that the most significant health problem among native Eskimos is diabetes. As we have seen in the previous chapter, one of the main contributing factors to the development of diabetes is having high blood glucose levels - being caused by a diet that has a *high glycemic load*. A high carbohydrate/low fat diet that contains grain based foods has a high glycemic load and causes blood glucose levels to rapidly increase after eating.

It is logical to suggest that native Eskimos are more susceptible to the adverse effects of a diet that has a high glycemic load. Their metabolisms have historically only had to deal with a very small amount of glucose. An Eskimos' body is not used to dealing with the rapid increase in blood glucose that is associated with a low fat / high carbohydrate diet – the diet that is recommended to them. It would take tens of thousands of years for them to adapt to this but it has been introduced suddenly in just a few decades.

North American Indians

American Indians suffer similar rates of obesity, diabetes and heart disease as do native Eskimos (4). The traditional diet of the American Indian was in many cases almost entirely made up of the wild animals of the case (1). This included: deer, buffalo, bear, moose, and fish. A small amount of plant food from berries, wild celery and corn was also eaten (7). When Dr Price visited the American Indians who were following their traditional way of life he was shown how they managed to keep themselves free from diseases such as scurvy.

When a moose was killed it was opened up at the back and two "balls of fat" just above the kidneys were taken out and cut up into small pieces. Each member of the family was then given a piece to eat. The Indians knew that eating a small amount of this part of the animal would prevent them from getting scurvy (1). The "balls of fat" were in fact the adrenal glands of the animal. We know through scientific research, that the adrenal glands provide one of the richest sources of vitamin C available from any food. The vitamin C available from the adrenal glands of the moose protected the American Indians from scurvy. The Indians had discovered this nutritional secret long before 'modern civilisation' had built laboratories to measure the nutrient content of foods.

American Indians are advised to reduce their fat intake, eat plenty of fruits and vegetables, eat low-fat cheese, skimmed milk, egg substitutes and soft margarines, and to cook with vegetable oils (7). Again, these guidelines represent a diet that is very different from their traditional diet – which included a large amount of protein and just a small amount of carbohydrate. The glycemic load of the traditional diet would be much lower than the diet that is now being recommended to American Indians. Increasing the glycemic load in this way, can only significantly increase the risk for diabetes and heart disease for these people.

In addition, low-fat foods that are more heavily processed such as low-fat cheese, skimmed milk and egg substitutes are not *whole foods* – they are denatured and low in vital nutrients. Where as the meats that was traditionally eaten were packed with life supporting nutrients. A lower intake of vital nutrients further increases the risk for disease. These nutrients are needed to protect the blood vessels and arteries from damage.

Australian Aborigines

Australian Aborigines are probably the oldest living race of people in the world (1). The traditional diet of the Aborigines depended on the district. Those who came from the coastal regions thrived on dugong, sea cow, shell fish and other types of sea food. This was supplemented with some sea plants. Where as people living in the interior districts thrived on land animals (such as kangaroo and wallaby), eggs, insects, leaves, berries, peas and roots (1).

Dr Price found that 'modern' nutrition was having a disastrous effect on Australian Aborigines. After consuming 'modern' foods for a relatively short period of time the fertility of these people had reduced to the point where the death rate far exceeded the birth rate. In summary, Dr Price wrote: "They demonstrate in a tragic way in inadequacy of the white man's dietary program" (1).

In the mid 1980s Professor Kerin O'Dea published an article in the journal *Diabetes* to document how a group of Australian Aborigines virtually recovered from diabetes in five weeks by returning to their traditional diet (8, 9).

Swiss – Loetschental Valley

At the time when Dr Price visited Switzerland, the most serious disease for the country as a whole was tuberculosis. However, the beautiful Loetschental Valley had not experienced a single case of this disease. The food here consisted mainly of rye bread and cheese. The cheese was eaten in slices as large as the slice of bread and it was made from the milk of cows that grazed on the grass near the snow line of the mountains. This cheese contained natural butter fat, which was the pride of the people and revered for its life-giving qualities. All of the dairy foods were unpasteurised and provided an excellent source of vitamins and minerals.

African Tribes

Although the Swiss of the Loetschental Valley thrived on a diet that contained a significant amount of grains (in the form of rye bread) certain African tribes have not fared so well. For in Africa, there appears to be a connection between the health of a particular group of people and the portion of the diet that is made up of grain based foods. Table 4A lists some of the African tribes that were studied by Dr Price. Generally, the tribes that consumed larger amounts of animal based foods were much more immune to dental cavities.

Amongst tribes who traditionally ate more foods of animal origin (which contained large amounts of saturated fat and cholesterol) it was not uncommon to find a complete absence of dental cavities. However, those tribes that extensively used cereal grains as food had around 6-7% of their teeth affected by dental cavities. It is widely accepted that dental health is a reliable indicator of nutritional status and general health. In addition, the tribes who consumed more animal based foods were generally physically stronger than those following a cereal or grain based diet.

Animal verses Plant Based Food

Researchers with an interest in the evolution of dietary habits and how this relates to health have investigated traditional diets around the world. They have found a huge variety in the composition of traditional diets. For example, the amount of meat that was eaten ranges from 270 grams to 1,400 grams per person per day (10). Figure 4A illustrates the composition of various traditional diets. It can be seen that the percentage of the diet that was made up of animal foods and plant based foods varied tremendously.

Although there is tremendous variation in traditional diets, it has also been revealed that:

Table 4A. Comparison of Some of the Tribes Studied by Dr Price.
Source: Reference (1).

Tribe	Main Foods Eaten	Dental Cavities (percentage of all teeth assessed)
Masai	Mostly raw milk, blood, and meat, with some vegetables and fruit.	0.4%.
Muhima	Mostly raw milk, blood, and meat.	0%
Maragoli	Large quantities of fish with some cereals and sweet potatoes.	0.2%
Baitu	Mostly dairy products from cattle and goats. Some sweet potatoes, cereals and bananas also eaten.	0%
Tribes living along the Nile River	Milk, blood and meat from cattle. Liver was a precious component of nutrition.	0%
Terrakeka	Fish and other animal foods	0%
Wanande	Bananas, sweet potatoes, cereals and goats' milk.	2.2%
Kikuyu	Sweet potatoes, corn, beans, bananas and millet	5.5%
Various Tribes in the Nyankunde Mission	Mostly cereals	6%
Various Tribes in the Bogora Mission	Mostly cereals, corn, and beans. Some sweet potatoes and bananas.	7.2%

- 73% of hunter-gatherer societies ate more animal foods than plant foods
- 14% of hunter-gatherer societies ate more plant foods than animal foods (11)

In fact, across all hunter-gatherer societies, the median consumption was around 66-75% animal foods and just 26-35% plant foods (11).

It is well established that human beings are omnivores: having the biological requirement to eat both animal and plant foods. However this data shows that animal foods would have been the preferred

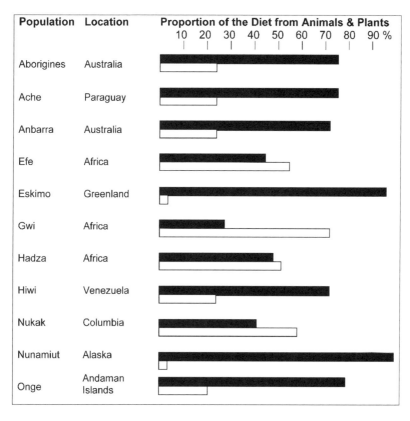

Figure 4A. The Amount of Animal Food verses Plant Food in Various Traditional Diets. Adapted from Reference (10) and (11).

energy source for the majority of worldwide hunter-gatherers (11).

In addition, 97% of the world's hunter-gatherers would have exceeded the fat intake that is recommended to people in the UK and America (11). Despite this, all hunter-gatherers were virtually free of heart disease.

These facts can help to explain why the UK and America, along with other countries, are experiencing a rapid increase in the incidence of diabetes. Genetically, a large proportion of humans are not able to cope with a high carbohydrate/low fat diet. As mentioned above, the high *glycemic load* of this diet results in high blood glucose levels that cause diabetes.

An evolutionary approach to nutrition can also help to explain why the trend towards a high carbohydrate/low fat diet corresponds with an increase in the rate of heart disease. Again, the main culprit being high blood glucose levels – which damage the walls of the arteries that supply blood and oxygen to the heart. Some of the mechanisms associated with this are discussed in chapter 12.

However, it would be inappropriate to suggest that diabetes and heart disease would be eliminated overnight by the ubiquitous adoption of a high protein diet. Since there are those people who do function best on a low fat / high carbohydrate diet. The challenge is to establish what proportion of carbohydrate, protein and fat suits each individual person.

The Two Laws of Nutrition

The work of Dr Price and numerous other researchers over the last century has been remarkably consistent and has revealed two fundamental laws of nutrition. These are:

1. Food is most nutritious in its natural state (as described in the appendix)
2. Each person has totally unique requirements for foods based on their genetic heritage and lifestyle. This applies to the macronutrients (carbohydrate, protein and fat) and to micronutrients (vitamins, minerals and trace elements).

These two simple rules should form the basis of any nutritional guidelines. If these laws are not obeyed, we can be absolutely certain that disease and degeneration will occur. Unfortunately nutritional advice in the 21st century is heavily influenced by politics and commercial interests. While this is the case, the general public will be subjected to a continuous deterioration in health.

Finding Your Own Nutritional Requirements

It is practically impossible to determine our own individual genetic heritage. In order to do this we would have to trace our family tree back for tens of thousands of years. We can however develop ways to measure how our individual metabolism is functioning today.

Rather than trying to find a simple set of nutritional recommendations to suit everyone, it makes much more sense to develop tools that enable individual people to determine their own individual requirements for foods. Thankfully, a range of these tools already exist. Dr Roger Williams, the great biochemist who discovered many of the *B vitamins*, said that at the metabolic level we are all as unique as we are in our fingerprints (12). Our metabolic individuality determines our individual nutritional requirements. This individuality permeates a number of different levels within the body. In order to understand each level it may be necessary to complete a range of metabolic tests.

The best tests we have available to us today are not genetic tests. Some scientists have attempted to create genetic tests but they are very much in their infancy. What we currently have are tests that measure how our genes are *expressing* themselves. We do not have to look deep into our DNA structure in order to understand our metabolism. Since our DNA expresses itself in a large number of ways that can be measured directly.

In fact, tools to measure how our genes are expressing themselves, rather than specific DNA tests, are probably always going to be more appropriate. Since our individual nutritional requirements are governed by not just our DNA but also our lifestyle habits over a period of time.

Of the tools we have readily available to us, the most widely adopted is a system called *Metabolic Typing™*. This system incorporates a range of different tests that are used to understand how an individual person's metabolism is currently functioning. Metabolic Typing™ has been influenced by a wide range of researchers over the last century, and the general principles date back to antiquity. However, during the last 30 years the process has been further developed and refined by William Wolcott, who is regarded as the worlds leading expert on the subject. William Wolcott has set up a company called *Healthexcel Inc.*, to assist health professionals in incorporating this health building system into their practice. He has also written an excellent book called *The Metabolic Typing Diet* (13).

One of the core benefits of Metabolic Typing™ is that it enables us to work out the basic proportions of carbohydrate, protein and fat that suits an individual person's metabolism. With this knowledge, we are much better able to control blood glucose levels and maintain optimum health. A full discussion of Metabolic Typing™ is beyond the scope of this book, however, in the broadest sense, an individual person can be a *carbohydrate type*, a *balanced type*, or a *protein type*. A carbohydrate type will require more carbohydrate in their diet and a protein type will require more protein and fat in their diet. Similarly, a balanced type requires roughly equal proportions of carbohydrate, protein and fat. This can be thought of in the context of a radio dial as illustrated in figure 4B, where each person can 'tune-in' to their own individual requirements.

Some readers will already be aware of Metabolic Typing™, and may already be working with a qualified Metabolic Typing

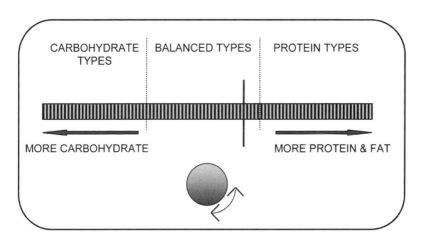

Figure 4B. Radio Dial Representation of Carbohydrate, Balanced and Protein Metabolic Types.

Practitioner. Other readers can obtain information about the range of programs available by logging on to the web resources for this book at: www.29billion.com.

CHAPTER 5

Cholesterol Causes Heart Disease: Impossible!

"Truth exists, only falsehood has to be invented"
Georges Braque

In December 1984 a panel of fourteen people met in Bethesda, Maryland for a Consensus Development Conference (1). This conference was organised by the American National Heart, Lung, and Blood Institute (NHLBI). The aim was to determine the relationship between cholesterol and heart disease. This was a significant event in both scale and importance. The audience included more than 600 physicians/researchers and the findings of the conference would have a great influence on the health advice that was to be given to the general public.

Once a consensus had been reached, a report of recommendations would be issued. However, the panel of people selected to prepare this report were carefully hand-picked by the NHLBI (2) and the guidelines that were subsequently published did not represent the view of many of the attendees.

The hypothesis was that as cholesterol levels rise, the risk for heart disease increases. Therefore, by lowering cholesterol levels we can reduce the risk for heart disease and reduce the number of people dieing of a heart attack. The 'evidence' was put forward, however, a number of researchers objected to the hypothesis.

Michael Oliver, a well respected heart expert, who was a past president of the Royal College of Physicians, had concerns. He explained that there was no benefit in lowering cholesterol because a reduction in deaths from heart disease is counter-acted by an increase in deaths from other causes (1).

Since the overall objective of cholesterol drugs is to save lives, it would not make any sense to prescribe a drug that potentially reduces the risk associated with heart disease, but at the same time, increases the risk of death from another cause. This is why it is important to look at the overall death rates associated with a clinical trial.

Other eminent researchers at the consensus conference did not agree with the cholesterol hypothesis (1-4). Despite this, the conclusion was in favour of it and a full scale national education program was launched to inform people about the dangers of cholesterol.

It has been suggested that this was not a consensus development meeting at all and the conclusion must have been decided upon before the conference took place (1, 4). Since there are questions about how the event proceeded. For example, the conference only lasted two and a half days, but more than 30 years of research had to be assessed before a conclusion could be reached. Printed copies of the plan for the new cholesterol education program were scheduled to be distributed at 8.30am the next morning and the program would be announced to the public during a scheduled press conference three hours later. It seems that the organisers were sufficiently confident of the outcome that they were able to schedule this press conference before the cholesterol hypothesis had been properly discussed.

Since 1984, billions of dollars have been spent on trying to prove the idea that cholesterol causes heart disease. However, all of these efforts have either failed to show any connection, or have been scientifically flawed. This will be discussed in more detail later in this chapter and the chapters that follow. First, it would be logical to include a very brief introduction to what we are told about cholesterol and how cholesterol is used within the body.

What We Are Told About Cholesterol

According to the British Heart Foundation (5), cholesterol is one of the most important risk factors for developing heart disease. It is stated that the risk increases as blood cholesterol levels increase. We are told that:

- Total cholesterol level should be below 5mmol/l[1]

- LDL (low density lipoprotein) is 'bad' cholesterol and this should be reduced to a level below 3mmol/l

- HDL (high density lipoprotein) is 'good' cholesterol and this should be above 1mmol/l

Then just to make it even more complicated, the total cholesterol level divided by the HDL level should be less than 4.5.

In addition, it is postulated that:

---

[1] Cholesterol is measured in millimoles per litre of blood, which is a molecular count and is abbreviated to mmol/l. Cholesterol is sometimes measured in milligrams per decilitre (by weight), abbreviated to mg/dl. To convert mmol/l of cholesterol to mg/dl multiply by 39.

- HDLs are 'good' cholesterol because they remove the unnecessary cholesterol from the blood stream and transport it back to the liver.

- Saturated fats cause cholesterol levels to increase.

What Is Cholesterol?

The human body is believed to be made up of around 100 trillion cells. It is very difficult for us to image this kind of number. If we equate one cell to one second in time and then countdown seconds (cells), by the time we had counted 100 trillion cells we would be 3.2 million years into the future!

Cholesterol is an integral and vital part of every single one of these cells. It forms the starting point for the synthesis of vitamin D, various hormones and bile acids for digestion. Cholesterol is also involved in the formation of synapses (6). Synapses allow nerve cells to communicate with each other. Therefore, a lack of cholesterol can lead to problems with the brain and nervous system.

So without sufficient cholesterol in the body there would be a deficiency of vital nutrients, inadequate digestion, a lack of hormones, and basically no chance what so ever that human life itself could exist.

There is still a great deal that we do not know about cholesterol and the way it works with other substances within the body. But one thing we can be certain of is that cholesterol is critically important for all life-supporting functions.

The Math Does Not Agree

Although we are constantly told that high cholesterol increases the risk for heart disease, the data we have available to us proves that mathematically this is impossible.

The measurement and recording of physical, biological and social data reveals that most things exhibit a *normal distribution* or *bell shaped curve*. This phenomenon has been observed for centuries. It is the most fundamental and the most widely used concept of statistical analysis. The bell curve has certain characteristics. For example, if we measure the height of the population in the UK, we would find that most people have an average height, a small number of people are very tall and a small number of people are very short. This is a normal distribution and is represented by the typical bell shaped curve.

As would be expected, the range of values that are found for cholesterol levels within a population also follow a normal distribution. This is represented in figure 5A, which shows that the distribution of cholesterol levels is symmetrical, in that:

- Most people have a cholesterol level that is close to the average value
- A few people have very high cholesterol levels
- A few people have very low cholesterol levels

The first point to mention is that the normal distribution for cholesterol levels has a wide range. Studies that included hundreds of thousands of people have shown that total cholesterol levels can vary from around 2.8 mmol/l to 8.8 mmol/l, even in healthy people who are free of heart disease (2). With such a wide range in values, it is difficult to establish a clear link between a specific level of cholesterol and risk for disease.

Cholesterol levels also change with age. They tend to increase during middle age and then decline in old age (2, 8). In addition, a wide range of other factors can affect the result of a cholesterol test. Dr Russell Smith (2) in his book *The Cholesterol Conspiracy* lists some of these other factors, which include:

- Body position
- Smoking or other nicotine use
- Stress
- Pain
- Fear
- Pregnancy
- Lack of exercise
- The use of various drugs and medicines
- Alcohol consumption
- How blood is drawn for the test
- The presence of hepatitis, gall bladder obstructions, low thyroid function etc

Blood cholesterol is also constantly changing and can be different depending on the season of the year (2).

Aside from the large variation in cholesterol levels and the difficulties in obtaining a reliable measurement, there are a number of fundamental questions that have so far been ignored. For example, the same distribution in total cholesterol levels that is seen in a healthy population is found in people who have heart disease.

If high cholesterol means that we are more likely to have heart disease, then the distribution of cholesterol levels for those people

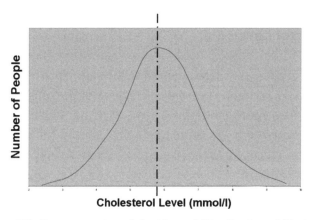

Figure 5A. Representation of the Normal Distribution of Cholesterol Levels. This distribution has been documented by Professor Brisson (7) and Dr Russell Smith (2).

who have heart disease must be different from those who not do have heart disease. However, this is not the case. The bell curve or normal distribution for people who do and who do not have heart disease is almost the same. This has been established from the analysis of large scale studies. It has been documented by Professor Brisson (7) using data from the Framingham Study, which is one of the largest studies ever done on cholesterol (9).

In addition, information published by the British Heart Foundation shows that 54% of people who die of heart disease have low cholesterol levels (10). Statistically, we are more likely to have heart disease if we have a lower cholesterol level. This is discussed further in chapter 7.

These facts can only mean that cholesterol is not a reliable indicator of heart disease risk, but the list of unanswered questions, paradoxes and contradictions does not stop there. Not by any means.

Most Heart Attacks Occur with Average Cholesterol Levels

Another paradox associated with the cholesterol idea is the fact that most people who have a heart attack have average cholesterol levels. This provides more evidence for the fact that cholesterol levels amongst people who have heart disease simply follow a normal distribution. Of course, if increasing cholesterol levels pose a risk for heart disease then most people who have a heart attack would have high cholesterol. But we have known for some time that they do not.

In the UK, the typical patient who has had a heart attack will have a total cholesterol level of around 6.0 mmol/l, which is the average cholesterol level for middle-aged and older people (11). The typical person who has a heart attack does not have substantially higher-than-average cholesterol (11).

A study published in the *Lancet*, one of the most respected medical journals in the world, included 5,754 patients from Australia and New Zealand who had already had a heart attack (12). The average total cholesterol level of this group of people was around 5.7 mmol/l. Data from the World Health Organisation *Global Infobase* (13, 14), shows that around the same time, the average cholesterol level for the general population was between 5.5 mmol/l and 5.8 mmol/l. People who had a heart attack had the same average cholesterol level as the general population.

A study published in the *American Journal of Cardiology* included 8,500 men with existing heart disease (15). The average total cholesterol level for this group of people was around 5.5 mmol/l, which (again, according to the World Health Organisation) is around the same or even slightly lower than the average cholesterol level for the general population (16).

No Cause for 'High' Cholesterol Has Been Found

If we believe what we are told about cholesterol, then high cholesterol is an urgent problem in many countries and this problem has reached epidemic proportions. For example, it is estimated that four million people in the UK are taking cholesterol lowering medication daily (17). As we shall see in subsequent chapters, there are a large number of additional people whom the pharmaceutical industry suggests should be taking these medications.

The obvious question to ask is where did this new disease (high cholesterol) that seems to afflict more people each day, actually come from, and what is causing so many people to be suffering from it?

As mentioned above, we are told that the main reason for having a high cholesterol level is eating too much saturated fat. Therefore, if cholesterol is such an urgent problem, we would expect that people in the UK are eating more saturated fat. However, this is not the case. As we have seen in chapter 2, the consumption of saturated fat in the UK has been decreasing. For example, the National Diet and Nutrition Survey (18) shows that between 1986 and 2000, the saturated fat intake of women aged 16 to 64 years in the UK reduced from 16.5% to 12.6%. This data is shown in table 5A.

The 'Experts' Contradict Themselves

So, according to the British Heart Foundation (BNF) the main cause of high cholesterol is eating too much saturated fat. However, on the BHF website, on a page describing cholesterol lowering medications, there are a series of questions and answers (19), one question asks:

Table 5A. Saturated Fat Intake (% of Total Energy) in the UK Source: National Diet and Nutrition Survey (18)

	Saturated Fat	
	MEN	WOMEN
1986/87	15.4%	16.5%
2000/01	12.6%	12.6%
DRV*	10%	

* DRV stands for 'Dietary Reference Value' and it is the estimated requirements for groups of people as specified by the British Nutrition Foundation.

"Can I lower my cholesterol level with a low fat diet?"

The answer that is given is:

"A good diet is one of the best ways to prevent ill health. However, on their own, dietary changes are not usually very effective at significantly lowering cholesterol."

So, eating saturated fat is the cause of high cholesterol, however reducing fat intake does not reduce cholesterol levels! At this point we should all be very worried indeed! In order to create a new disease you have to find a cause but when that cause is found not to exist, you have a problem. The supporters of the cholesterol idea have dealt with this problem in the same way that they have dealt with the many other fundamental paradoxes and contradictions - by simply ignoring it.

What Are LDLs and HDLs?

If LDL 'cholesterol' is bad and HDL 'cholesterol' is good, then what is the difference between them? Actually, the difference between LDLs and HDLs has got nothing to do with cholesterol. This is because LDLs and HDLs are not really cholesterol at all! Dr Malcolm Kendrick in his book *The Great Cholesterol Con* (20) explains this fact very well.

Cholesterol does not mix with water; therefore in order for it to be transported through the blood stream it has to be carried inside something called a *lipoprotein*. A lipoprotein is a kind of bundle of fats, protein, and other substances that moves around the body. Lipoproteins carry a number of very important substances that are needed by the body's cells. A pictorial view of a lipoprotein is shown in figure 5B. LDLs and HDLs are the lipoproteins that carry cholesterol.

Often, after a cholesterol test, people are told something like "you have slightly high cholesterol but it's ok because your 'good' cholesterol is also high" or "your 'bad' cholesterol is too high and we need to reduce it". These statements are totally meaningless because LDLs and HDLs carry the same cholesterol molecule. The structure of cholesterol is illustrated in figure 5C. This molecule is the same weather it happens to be in a LDL or a HDL.

The difference between a high density lipoprotein (HDL) and a low density lipoprotein (LDL) is their relative size. HDLs are smaller than LDLs.

The False Idea of 'Good' and 'Bad' Cholesterol

Over the years the cholesterol idea has gone through a number of dramatic changes. The latest version of cholesterol theory is very different from the original hypothesis. None of the versions of the idea have been supported by the scientific studies. Therefore the

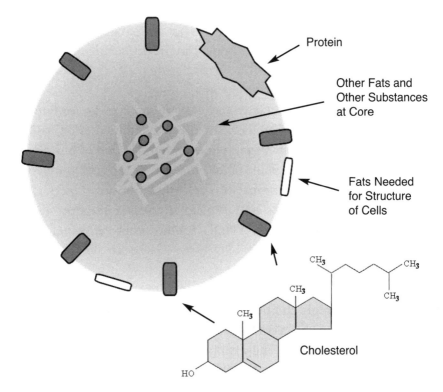

Protein

Other Fats and
Other Substances
at Core

Fats Needed
for Structure
of Cells

CH₃

Cholesterol

Figure 5B. The Basic Structure of a Lipoprotein

Figure 5C. Molecular Structure of Cholesterol

hypothesis has been repeatedly altered in anyway that will enable it to be kept alive.

The original idea stated that high cholesterol levels increase the risk for heart disease. However in February 1992, the American National Institutes of Health met for another 'Consensus Conference' because a problem had arisen with this hypothesis. Large numbers of people with low cholesterol levels were having heart attacks! (3) In response to this problem it was recommended that doctors should test for not just total cholesterol levels but also HDL ('good') levels and LDL ('bad') levels. Objections were raised to this by Dr Stephen Hulley of the University of California, who stated that this would lead to large numbers of low-risk people taking cholesterol-lowering drugs, which has been shown to increase overall death rates (3).

In the same way as the original 'Consensus Conference', valid objections seem to have been ignored. Since the cholesterol idea was modified in accordance with this illusion of 'good' and 'bad' types of cholesterol. Now, the people who support the cholesterol idea have a number of different ways that they can suggest someone has a problem with cholesterol. Previously, a person would only be a candidate for cholesterol drugs if they had high total cholesterol. But now, they can also be a potential candidate if they have high 'bad' cholesterol, or if they have low levels of 'good' cholesterol, or if the level of 'good' cholesterol is low compared with total cholesterol, and so on.

The modification of the idea to include 'good' and 'bad' cholesterol not only gets the supporters of the hypothesis out of a tricky situation (the lack of evidence to support their hypothesis), but it also gives them more possibilities to suggest that someone needs to take cholesterol drugs. It also significantly complicates the issue and makes it more difficult for people to raise objections to their hypothesis.

The explanation we are given for HDLs being 'good' and LDLs being 'bad' is related to the direction of travel that these molecules follow within the body. Dr Uffe Ravnskov, a researcher from Sweden, describes LDLs and HDLs as acting like microscopic submarines (21). This is a useful analogy. Most of the cholesterol in the body is made in the liver. The LDL 'submarines' transport cholesterol from the liver to the cells, including those cells in the walls of arteries. The HDL 'submarines' transport cholesterol back to the liver.

At first appearance, it may seem logical to suggest that LDLs are bad because they transport cholesterol to artery walls. However, we have to keep in mind that this action simply provides a normal and vitally important function. As stated above, all cells within the body need cholesterol. It is cholesterol that makes cells waterproof. Cells need to be waterproof in order for the internal structure of the cell to be protected from the external environment. Therefore, a mechanism is required that enables all the cells to get the cholesterol they critically need. LDLs provide this important function.

Cholesterol is an interesting molecule. It is often called a fat, but chemically it should be called an alcohol, although it does not behave like alcohol (21). The integrate structure of cholesterol provides the protection needed for cells.

When cells become damaged, they need cholesterol to repair themselves. A discussion of the tissue repair qualities of cholesterol can be found in the scientific literature at least as far back as 1975 (22, 23). However, this important issue is conveniently ignored by those who support the idea of good and bad cholesterol.

There are a large number of reasons why the cells within the walls of the arteries that supply blood and oxygen to the heart may become damaged. For example, smoking cigarettes, high blood glucose (sugar) levels, high stress, and toxicity can cause this type of damage to the arteries. In response to this, the body may need to make more cholesterol, which it sends to the cells that need it via LDL submarines. The LDL submarines may be required in greater numbers in order to perform this function more efficiently. But this is the effect of the initial damage to the cells and not the cause.

Some researchers have stated that there is a mathematical link to show that the level of LDL submarines increases in some people who have heart disease. However, even if some studies do show this, it is wrong to just assume that LDLs cause heart disease. Especially if we consider the latest understanding of how heart disease develops. This is discussed in more detail in chapter 11.

Suggesting that LDLs cause heart disease is like blaming the traffic police at the scene of a motor vehicle accident. Yes, the police are there, but to clear up the incident; not as the cause of the accident.

CHAPTER 6

Dietary Cholesterol and Saturated Fat

*"A belief is not merely an idea the mind possesses; it is an idea
that possesses the mind"*
Robert Oxton Bolt

Dietary cholesterol and saturated fat are routinely labelled as "artery clogging". People are led to believe that eating foods containing these substances will lead to an early grave. Many readers will be surprised to learn that this notion is nothing more than a belief that has never been proven. When we repeatedly hear that these foods cause heart disease, we assume that scientists have actually done experiments that clearly demonstrate how this happens. The fact is that any experiments that have been done have either been inconclusive or have actually proved the opposite to be true.

This chapter specifically looks at dietary cholesterol and saturated fats in terms of what we have been brainwashed to believe about them. Throughout the discussion, it has been necessary to make reference to LDLs as 'good' cholesterol and HDLs as 'bad' cholesterol. Whether or not these are indeed 'good' and 'bad' respectively is a separate issue. The aim here is to simply show that what we have been told about the effects of dietary cholesterol and saturated fat is completely wrong.

Dietary Cholesterol

During the early days, supporters of the cholesterol idea believed that eating cholesterol caused the level of cholesterol in the blood stream to increase. The report that was widely circulated after the Consensus Development Conference in 1984 (1) recommended that dietary cholesterol intake should be limited to 250 - 300mg per day. This constitutes roughly the same amount of cholesterol found in one egg.

These recommendations formed part of the Cholesterol Education Program and despite the fact that many doctors and researchers at the time did not agree, the idea became very popular.

One of the more widespread suggestions, connected with this fear of dietary cholesterol was that it would be healthier to separate egg whites from the yoke. Since it is the yoke of an egg that contains the cholesterol, some 'experts' thought that just eating the egg white would provide a good source of protein without the need to consume the 'dangerous' cholesterol. This idea became popular with bodybuilders and some health and fitness magazines jumped on the bandwagon to popularise the idea.

The egg is one of the most nutritious and well-balanced foods available. It is the very symbol of life and if it contains a high level of cholesterol, then this must surely tell us something about the need for cholesterol within the body. Why would nature create something that is only fit for consumption when 'experts' have decided to hack-out half of its structure?

There are numerous examples that contradict the idea that eating cholesterol causes blood cholesterol levels to increase. For example, the famous Masai tribe of East Africa traditionally eat large amounts of cholesterol and yet their blood cholesterol levels remain low (2).

After the Cholesterol Education Program was distributed, large scale studies were published contradicting the idea that dietary cholesterol should be avoided. These studies showed no relationship between dietary cholesterol and cholesterol levels in the blood. As a result, even the strongest supporters of the cholesterol idea had to admit that the actual consumption of cholesterol has got nothing at all to do with blood cholesterol levels.

The latest UK National Diet and Nutrition Survey, states that "dietary cholesterol has a relatively small and variable effect" on blood cholesterol levels (3). It also states that the Committee on Medical Aspects of Food and Nutrition Policy (COMA), the group who set recommended daily amounts of nutrients for people in the UK, have not set any value for cholesterol consumption.

However the National Diet and Nutrition Survey does quote another report (4), suggesting that cholesterol intake should not exceed 1992 consumption levels of 245mg. Unfortunately, the survey does not mention that this report is outdated since it states that "dietary cholesterol can significantly increase blood cholesterol". Another report involving the World Health Organisation makes the vague suggestion that "reasonable restriction of dietary cholesterol (less than 300 mg per day) is advised" (5).

There is no scientific foundation for a suggested maximum cholesterol intake of 245mg or 300mg. There is not one single scientific reference to support this recommendation. It is a number that is simply pulled out of thin air.

Unfortunately there are a large number of organisations within the food and pharmaceutical industries that benefit from keeping this misconception alive. The fact that more has not been done to educate the public about this issue is testament to the power and control that these organisations have over the information that consumers receive.

We know that the liver and the intestines make cholesterol in accordance with what the body needs. Cholesterol levels in the blood are influenced by a large number of factors and (as with everything) there are considerable differences between different people. One thing we do know for sure is that the body can make cholesterol from not just fat, but protein and carbohydrate as well. Cholesterol is so important that the body has definite pathways to make it from just about anything.

In addition to there being no evidence for a link between dietary cholesterol and cholesterol levels in the blood stream, there is also no evidence linking the cholesterol that we eat with heart disease.

If cholesterol in our food causes heart disease, then logic suggests that patients who have heart disease would have eaten more cholesterol than people who do not suffer with heart disease.

Dr Uffe Ravnskov (6) has completed an analysis of ten studies that recorded cholesterol consumption and heart disease. In some studies the patients with heart disease had eaten slightly more cholesterol; however in other studies it was the people who did not have heart disease who ate more cholesterol. In fact, overall, when the data from all the studies are combined, cholesterol consumption was slightly higher amongst people without heart disease.

Saturated Fat and Blood Cholesterol

As discussed in the previous chapter, the British Heart Foundation cites saturated fat as the main cause of high cholesterol in the UK A similar statement is made by the National Heart, Lung and Blood Institute in America. Again, readers may be surprised to learn that the alleged link between dietary saturated fat and high cholesterol levels in the blood has also never been proven.

This misconception started with Dr Ancel Keys. Dr Keys was very keen to point out that average blood cholesterol levels are high in countries that eat lots of foods containing saturated fat. In 1958 he described this 'connection' by plotting the data for various countries on a graph. He attempted to show, as the consumption of fat increases so does the average cholesterol level (7).

However, just in the same way as other published work by Keys, he had omitted critical data from the graph in order to support his idea. It is now well known in the scientific community that at the time Keys published his paper, data was available for additional countries that did not appear on his graph, and if these countries were included, the data would have shown no connection at all between fat intake and blood cholesterol levels.

One of the largest studies ever done on this subject was the Framingham Heart Study. This study began in 1948 and involved around 6,000 people from the town of Framingham in Massachusetts. The people in the study were split into two groups – those who consumed a large amount of cholesterol and saturated fat and those who consumed small amounts. As discussed by Sally Fallon and Mary Enig in their book *Nourishing Traditions* (8), forty years in to the study, its director, Dr. William Castelli, had to admit; "In Framingham, the more saturated fat one ate, the more cholesterol one ate, the lower the person's serum cholesterol". In this highly significant study, it was shown that eating saturated fat and cholesterol actually lowered blood cholesterol levels.

There are countless other studies that completely contradict the idea saturated fat causes cholesterol levels to increase. Other authors have dealt with this subject in great detail (6, 8, 9, 10). Faced with a huge body of evidence against their hypothesis, the supporters of the cholesterol idea found themselves in a tricky situation. True to form, the cholesterol proponents were able to think of another modification to their idea that would breathe life into it for a few more years.

The new version of the cholesterol idea states that it is not blood cholesterol in general that is increased by saturated fat in the diet, but more specifically, it is LDLs (the so called 'bad' cholesterol) that are increased by eating saturated fat.

The idea that saturated fat increases the number of LDLs came from studies that were done on animals. During one study, hamsters were fed high doses of saturated fat and it was found that this correlated with an increase in blood LDLs (11). Most people know that hamsters normally eat seeds, grains, nuts, and vegetables. Feeding a vegetarian hamster saturated fat, which it does not have the metabolic machinery to deal with, will undoubtedly have adverse effects. The hamster is not designed to metabolise saturated fats. This experimental diet may have caused tissue damage in the hamster's body. The natural response to this may be to make more cholesterol in an attempt to improve cellular integrity and lessen the damage.

If the foods that were fed to the hamster contained significant amounts of cholesterol, which of course they probably did, this would have accounted for another possible explanation. Not because there is anything inherently bad about cholesterol, but because vegetarian animals are not adapted to eliminating large amounts of cholesterol from their bodies (12).

Even if we accept these ill found animal experiments, there is strong evidence showing that saturated fats do not increase LDLs, and this evidence is based on studies with people: not vegetarian animals.

A study that was published in the *Lancet* looked at data collected during the UK National Diet and Nutrition Survey (13). This study included 1420 people. The researchers found no connection between saturated fat and the level of LDLs. No connected was also found between saturated fat and total cholesterol levels.

A study published in *The New England Journal of Medicine* (14) compared the effects of a low fat (conventional) diet with a high fat diet. The people who took part in the study were split into two groups respectively. The people in the high fat diet group were asked to follow the *Atkins' Diet* (15), which advocates large amounts of saturated fats from animal proteins.

After one year, each group was assessed for risk factors associated with heart disease. It was found that there was no significant difference in total cholesterol levels or LDL ('bad' cholesterol) levels between the two groups. In addition, the group following the high fat Atkins' Diet showed a significant increase in HDL ('good' cholesterol) levels, throughout the entire study period. The people who ate the most foods high in saturated fat showed the most reduction in risk for heart disease.

In 2008, a similar study was published in *The New England Journal of Medicine*. In this study three different diets were compared (a low carbohydrate / Atkins' type diet, a Mediterranean type diet, and a low fat diet) and this time the trial ran for two years. Again, the researchers found no link between increasing the amount of saturated fat in the diet and LDL levels (16). As with the study mentioned above, the diet that contained the most saturated fat produced the best overall results in terms of risk for heart disease.

Another study compared a low fat diet with a high fat diet in women who are overweight but otherwise healthy (17). Again the people in the study were split into two groups. One group followed a low fat diet and the other group followed a high fat diet. At the end of the six month study, cholesterol levels were measured, and there were no significant differences between the two groups. The people in the high fat diet group had eaten twice as much saturated fat, yet their total cholesterol was unchanged, their LDL levels were unaffected and their 'good' cholesterol (HDLs) had increased slightly. The results observed in the high fat diet group were the opposite of what we should expect if we believe the supporters of the cholesterol idea. The authors of the study stated "This study provides a surprising challenge to prevailing dietary practice".

In another study a low carbohydrate diet was compared with a low fat conventional diet (18). The people in the low carbohydrate diet group were instructed not to eat more than 30g of carbohydrate per day (just slightly more than is allowed on the Atkins' Diet). The majority of the food eaten in the low carbohydrate group would have contained large amounts of saturated fat. At the end of the one year follow up, changes in both total cholesterol and LDLs were not significantly different between the groups. In addition, so called 'good' cholesterol

(HDLs) had decreased more in people who followed the conventional diet that was low in fat.

Yet another study compared the effects of low fat and high fat diets (19). In this study the people in the low fat diet group were instructed not to eat more than 10 percent saturated fat. The people in the high fat diet group were allowed to eat as much saturated fat as they liked and unlimited eggs. The level of LDLs did not differ statistically when the results were compared. The most significant different between the two groups was that the high fat diet provided an increase in 'good' cholesterol (HDLs).

It is worth mentioning one more study that was published in the *Journal of the American Medical Association* (20). This study compared four weight loss diets representing a spectrum of low to high fat and carbohydrate intakes. The diet which had the highest saturated fat intake, rather than producing adverse effects, showed the most favourable effects - this group of people (who ate the most saturated fat) again showed the greatest reduction in risk for heart disease.

As we can see there are numerous studies to show that saturated fat does not cause LDLs to increase. The evidence actually shows that LDLs are unaffected by saturated fat and diets that are low in saturated fat cause levels of 'good' cholesterol to decrease.

Some 'expects' suggest that longer studies need to be done before we can be sure that saturated fat does not have adverse effects on cholesterol levels. However, these people could be accused of having double standards, since some of the studies that are supposed to show adverse effects of saturated fats, such as the animal experiment mentioned above were just thirty days in duration.

There are also studies that have looked at not just cholesterol levels but the actual incidence of heart disease, in the context of different amounts of saturated fat in the diet. For example, a study published in the *American Journal of Clinical Nutrition* included 75,521 women, who were followed for 10 years in order to determine the effects of different diets (21). The primary aim of the study was to determine the effect of increasing the *glycemic load* of the diet, but the amount of saturated fat was also recorded. The women in the group that ate the lowest amount of saturated fat had 186 cases of heart disease; where as those with the highest amount of saturated fat intake had 139 cases. This study shows that saturated fat is involved in heart disease: not as a cause of the disease, but rather, as a protective influence.

Researchers from Harvard University investigated the effects of different diets on the progression of heart disease. 235 women who already had heart disease were included in their study. The women were followed for around 3 years. Just in the same way as the studies mentioned above, the researchers found that saturated fat was not related to LDL 'cholesterol'. They also found that greater saturated fat intake was associated with less progression of heart disease. Where as, polyunsaturated fat and carbohydrate intakes were associated with a greater progression of heart disease (22).

We can see from the evidence presented in this chapter that dietary saturated fat and cholesterol do not affect blood cholesterol levels in the way that we are led to believe. Neither do they cause heart disease.

Our body's response to different types of foods depends on our individual makeup and genetic heritage. Just how much saturated fat or any other nutrient an individual person requires is a matter of biochemical individuality.

CHAPTER 7

Lowering Cholesterol – Is it a Good Idea?

"I do not believe today everything I believed yesterday; I wonder will I believe tomorrow everything I believe today"
Matthew Arnold

Here in the UK a great deal of effort has been directed towards 'educating' the general public about the 'dangers' associated with cholesterol. It is fair to say that this message has reached most adults and the supporters of the cholesterol idea have been very successful in creating a fear of cholesterol. This has been reinforced with television advertisements using shock tactics in an attempt to encourage more people to pay attention to the cholesterol message. It almost seems as if people have been made to fear cholesterol more than heart disease itself.

We are led to believe that average cholesterol levels are too high in the UK, or cholesterol levels have substantially risen within the UK. The message we receive is that cholesterol is an urgent problem which needs to be addressed if we are going to reduce the number of people who suffer with heart disease: the most common cause of death in the UK.

Direct statements about historical trends in blood cholesterol levels are seldom made. However, the hype surrounding cholesterol creates a suggestion that cholesterol levels have increased during recent years. Why else would cholesterol be such a problem? Why else do so many people need to take cholesterol lowering medications? Surely this is because average cholesterol levels have risen?

In fact, it is quite difficult to find data associated with past cholesterol levels in the UK. The British Heart Foundation statistics website (www.heartstats.org) publishes an extremely wide range of data and statistics on heart disease but does not publish information about average cholesterol levels for previous years. This is a pity because this data would be interesting to see.

The World Health Organisation *Global InfoBase* (1) contains cholesterol data on most countries around the world. Comparing the data available for 1998 in this database with data published by the Department of Health (2), average cholesterol levels for adults in the UK remained unchanged until 2003 at around 5.5mmol/l (millimoles per litre). However more recent estimates have suggested that the national average has dropped to 5.1mmol/l (3).

Data is published, concerning the incidence of 'high' cholesterol during previous years. Overall, in England and Scotland, for both men and women, the number of people with 'high' cholesterol was lower in 2003 than it was in 1994. The trend during this time period was different for different age groups. For some age groups, there was a decrease between 1994 and 1998 and then an increase in 2003. However, in a number of age groups there has been a steady decrease since 1994 (3). For example, table 7A shows the percentage of men in England between the ages of 65 and 74 who had a total cholesterol level above 5.0mmol/l. In this age group, between 1994 and 2003, the percentage dropped from around 87% to 68%.

Table 7A. Percentage of Men in England between 65 and 74 Years Old Who Have a Total Cholesterol Level Equal to or Above 5.0mmol/l, in 1994, 1998 and 2003.

Year	Percentage of Men with Total Cholesterol Level Equal to or Above 5.0 mmol/l
1994	87.4
1998	76.0
2003	68.8

If the number of people with 'high' cholesterol is actually decreasing, why then, we might ask, are the numbers of people who take cholesterol lowering drugs rapidly increasing? Cholesterol lowering medications belong to a group of medications known as *lipid regulating drugs* or *lipid lowering drugs*. The use of which has increased rapidly since the mid-1990s, and increased sixteen fold in the last decade (4).This is shown in figure 7A.

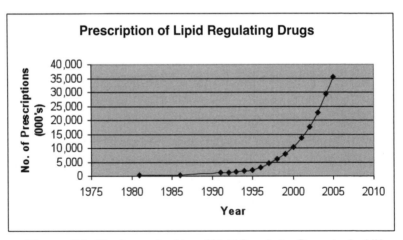

Figure 7A. The Increasing Use of Lipid Regulating Drugs in the UK
Source: British Heart Foundation (www.heartstats.org)

Supporters of the cholesterol idea might suggest that the reduction in cholesterol levels is due to this rapid increase in the number of people taking cholesterol lowering medications. While this would have some effect on some age groups, there are a number of reasons why it is not possible for these drugs to account for the overall reduction. For example, while average cholesterol levels in the UK remained the same between 1998 and 2003, the use of cholesterol lowering medications increased exponentially. Also, the percentage of 16 to 24 year old men in England with 'high' cholesterol reduced from 32.4% in 1994 to 22.5% in 1998 (3) – a reduction of around 10%. Since 16 to 24 year olds were generally not considered candidates for cholesterol lowering drugs during this time, it is impossible for the drugs to be responsible for this reduction.

Readers will recall from chapter 2 that the consumption of saturated fat has reduced in the UK Supports of the cholesterol idea may suggest that this reduction in the amount of saturated fat in the diet is responsible for any reduction in average cholesterol levels. However, we have already seen in the previous chapter that there is a large body of evidence to prove that saturated fat intake does not affect blood cholesterol levels.

The reality is: if cholesterol levels have reduced in the UK, we do not yet know why this has happened. The misplaced cholesterol phobia has prevented investigation into this. The main point to be made here is that there is no evidence that cholesterol levels in the UK are increasing and no justification for creating a feeling of panic about cholesterol.

So if cholesterol levels have not risen in the UK, we must assume that the average cholesterol level is high when compared with other countries. In fact, the British Heart Foundation (BHF) is always very keen to point out that the average cholesterol level in the UK is high by international standards. The BHF and other supporters of the cholesterol idea often use the example of China for comparison with the UK.

It is true that average cholesterol levels are lower in China. However, comparisons with China do not give a balanced view, since China has one of the lowest average cholesterol levels in the world. There are also many countries that have a higher level of cholesterol than the UK. Across the world, there is a huge variation in cholesterol levels. As yet, we do not know if this has any significance.

Professor Peter Weissberg, Medical Director at the BHF has stated: "Research undertaken around the world tells us that the lower your cholesterol level is, the lower your risk of a heart attack" (5). This statement by Professor Weissberg is at odds with the data we have available to us and the data that is published by the BHF itself. There are numerous examples of countries where the cholesterol level is 'high' but the rate of heart disease is low - completely contradicting the cholesterol idea. This is discussed in the next section below.

Cholesterol and Heart Disease: a Global Perspective

The BHF publishes information about the rate of heart attacks around the world. Much of this data is based on the World Health Organisation *MONICA* project (6) and is summarised in figure 7B. This data shows that the UK populations studied have almost the highest rates of heart attacks in the world.

If high cholesterol is a significant risk factor for having a heart

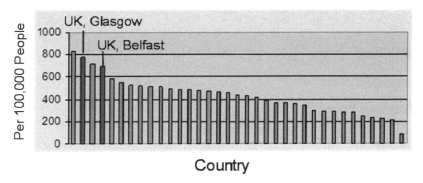

Figure 7B. Comparison of the Rate of Heart Attacks in Various Populations Surveyed in the World Health Organisation MONICA Project (Men Aged 35–64).

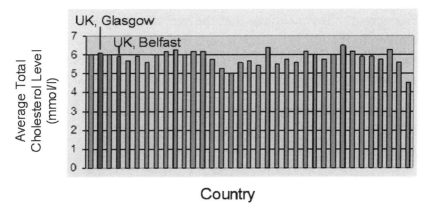

Figure 7C. Comparison of Average Cholesterol Levels in Populations Surveyed in the World Health Organisation MONICA Project. (Men Aged 35–64). Countries are listed in the same order as in figure 7B.

attack, we would expect that the countries that have the most heart attacks will also have the highest cholesterol levels. Figure 7C shows the average cholesterol level for the same countries listed in figure 7B. The countries are listed in the same order in both charts, so that we can compare the data. It can easily be seen that whilst a few countries have both higher cholesterol and a higher rate of heart attacks, most countries do not follow this pattern at all.

Around Europe

Similarly, within Europe there is no correlation between cholesterol levels and heart attacks. Using data available from the World Health Organisation *Global InfoBase* Country Comparison (7), we can compare the average cholesterol levels for various European countries. Figure 7D shows this data for women.

From figure 7D we can see that the average cholesterol level for women in the UK is the 12th lowest on a scale of 45 countries. A similar pattern is found for men in the UK, who are the 15th lowest on the same scale of 45 countries. So cholesterol levels are actually

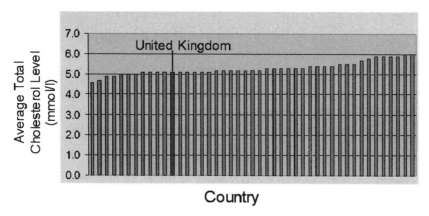

Figure 7D. Comparison of Average Total Cholesterol Levels (Women Aged 15 and Above) for Various European Countries. Source: World Health Organisation Global InfoBase Country Comparison

quite low when compared with the rest of Europe. Despite the fact that the UK has one of the highest rates of heart attacks in the world.

A large number of case studies within Europe contradict the idea that raised cholesterol causes people to have heart attacks. For example, in Ticino, Switzerland; men aged 35 to 64, have the highest cholesterol levels of all regions studied in the World Health Organisation MONICA project. The region has the highest percentage of men with high cholesterol levels above 7.8mmol/l. They eat more saturated fat than men in the UK. Yet they have one of the lowest rates of heart attacks.

In Moscow, Russia, men aged 35 to 64, have a moderate cholesterol level with one of the lowest rates of high cholesterol. They consume about half the amount of saturated fat as men in Ticino, but they have a much higher rate of heart attacks.

Men in Glasgow, UK have lower cholesterol levels than men in Ticino, but their rate of heart attacks is more than two and half times greater. As shown in table 7B and 7C.

A number of British health societies have recommended an ideal total cholesterol level of 4mmol/l for people in the UK who are classified as having a high risk for heart disease (8). This would be a very low level of cholesterol and it is not common in Europe or around the rest of the World. For example the global average for men is around 5mmol/l (9).

Cholesterol Levels Reduce: Heart Disease Increases

In England, the rate of heart disease is increasing in most age groups for both men and women. This is more apparent in older

Table 7B. Comparison of Cholesterol Levels and Rate of Heart Attacks for Men Aged 35-64 in Various Countries. Source: British Heart Foundation (www.heartstats.org)

	Switzerland, Ticino	Russia, Moscow	UK, Glasgow
Average Total Cholesterol (mmol/l)	6.5	5.3	6.1
% of Men with Cholesterol Level Above 7.8mmol/l	15	2	6
Rate of Heart Attacks (per 100,000)	290	477	777

Table 7C. Comparison of the Saturated Fat Intake of Switzerland, Russia and the United Kingdom, 1998. Source: British Heart Foundation (www.heartstats.org)

	Switzerland	Russia	UK
% of Total Energy From Saturated Fat	15.3	8.3	13.5

age groups, particularly in people aged 75 years and above (10).

It is interesting that whilst older age groups have experienced the largest increase in heart disease, they have also experienced the largest reduction in total cholesterol levels. If higher cholesterol levels are associated with a greater risk for heart disease we would, of course, expect the incidence of heart disease to reduce as the percentage of people with 'high' cholesterol reduces. However the opposite is true - between 1994 and 2003 the number of men aged 75 and above, having 'high' cholesterol decreased from 79% to 63%: at the same time the incidence of heart disease for this group increased from 22.7% to 26.4%. This is shown in table 7D.

In fact, it can also be seen from table 7D that, for men of all age

Table 7D. Comparison of the Incidence of Coronary Heart Disease and Percentage of Men with 'High' Cholesterol in England, between 1994 and 2003, for Various Age Groups. High Cholesterol is Designated as Equal to or Above 5mmol/l.
Source: British Heart Foundation (3, 10).

	% People with Coronary Heart Disease	% People with High Cholesterol
Men Aged 35-44		
1994	0.5	82
2003	0.9	77.3
Men Aged 45-54		
1994	3	88.3
2003	3.5	81.6
Men Aged 55-64		
1994	10.3	89.9
2003	11.1	80.5
Men Aged 65-74		
1994	21	87.4
2003	21.5	68.8
Men Aged 75+		
1994	22.7	79.4
2003	26.4	63.4

groups, as the percentage of those with 'high' cholesterol decreases, the number of men with heart disease increases. Similar trends are also found for a number of age groups in women (3,10).

This data, published by the BHF, shows that for almost all age groups in England, for both men and women, the incidence of heart disease has increased as cholesterol levels have decreased.

The Benefits of High Cholesterol

There is evidence that high cholesterol in elderly people is associated with a longer life. This was the conclusion of a study completed by a team of researchers at Yale University School of Medicine (11). Researchers in the Netherlands also found that in the case of the very elderly, life expectancy increases when cholesterol levels are higher. Those with higher cholesterol levels appeared to be better protected from cancer and infection (12).

A large number of studies have also shown high cholesterol to be protective in elderly people with heart failure (13 - 18). An article published in the *Lancet* proposed that in patients with heart failure lowering cholesterol levels is detrimental and higher levels of total cholesterol are beneficial (19).

Further evidence that higher cholesterol protects against infection was established by Professor Jacobs and Dr. Carlos Iribarren who followed more than 100,000 healthy individuals in the San Francisco area for fifteen years. At the end of the study those who had low cholesterol at the start of the study had a higher rate of infectious disease (20).

Another study published in the *Lancet*, looked at cholesterol levels and death rates in more than 3500 elderly Japanese/American men over a twenty year period. The authors of this paper confirmed what was found in previous studies – an increase in death rates in people with low blood cholesterol levels. The authors went on to say that not only do these results provide more evidence that low cholesterol in the elderly is associated with an increased risk of death, but they also suggest that people who have low cholesterol maintained over a twenty year period have the worst outlook for mortality (21).

Higher levels of cholesterol may also protect against Parkinson's disease. A study published in the journal *Movement Disorders* found that people with Parkinson's disease had lower LDL (so called 'bad' cholesterol) levels than people who did not have the disease (22).

We are told that high cholesterol represents a major risk factor for heart disease. The BHF states that 46% of people under 75 years of age in the UK who die from heart disease have high cholesterol (23). The World Health Organisation has stated that 60% of all coronary heart disease in developed countries is due to cholesterol levels above 3.8mmol/l (24). When you read these statements, at first glance, it might seem that cholesterol really is a major risk factor: however this data is actually telling us something quite different.

If 46% of people in the UK who have died of heart disease had high cholesterol, obviously this means that more than half of the people who die of heart disease do not have high cholesterol: which means of course that having a lower cholesterol level is associated with a greater chance of dieing from heart disease.

In a similar way, if 60% of people with heart disease have cholesterol levels above 3.8mmol/l, this means that 40% of heart disease is associated with cholesterol levels below 3.8mmol/l.

This may not seem very significant until we recall that the global average cholesterol level, for example in men, is around 5.0mmol/l (9). It is misleading to use a value of 3.8mmol/l as the reference point since this is a very low level of cholesterol. The fact that 40% of heart disease is associated with a cholesterol level below 3.8mmol/l disproves the idea that raised cholesterol causes heart disease – It certainly does not support the cholesterol idea!

Some people may respond to this data by suggesting that it is necessary to look at other risk factors along with cholesterol. Yes, it is. However, it is important to compare cholesterol levels in the way discussed above because this is exactly the same way that the whole cholesterol idea has been built. No physical evidence has been provided to demonstrate how having a raised cholesterol level in the blood causes heart disease. The so called 'evidence' has always been based on simple mathematical relationships such as the comparison of cholesterol levels with the rate of heart disease. It is easy to see that these suggested mathematical links are false.

A study published in the *Journal of the American Medical Association* analysed data for 122,458 patients enrolled in 14 international clinical trials (25). The authors compared the frequency of various risk factors in people who have had heart disease. They found that only 39% of all men and 34% of all women who had heart disease had high cholesterol or high triglycerides. If cholesterol was assessed independently of triglycerides this percentage may have been even less. If we look at the data provided in this study for different age groups we can also see that just 20% of men aged 75 years and above with heart disease had high cholesterol. Again, suggesting that people are more likely to have heart disease if they have low cholesterol.

Smarter People Have Higher Cholesterol

Researchers at Boston University investigated the relationship between total cholesterol levels and cognitive performance in 789 men and 1105 women (26). They discovered that low cholesterol levels were associated with a lower performance in tests for word fluency, attention/concentration, and overall cognitive performance.

Does Higher Cholesterol Protect Against Diabetes?

From chapter 2 we already know that the number of people with diabetes in the UK is rapidly increasing, and that diabetes poses a major risk for having cardiovascular disease (any problem with the heart or blood vessels). Yet, in the UK, people with diabetes tend to have lower cholesterol levels than the rest of the population.

In a study completed in Tayside, published in 1999, 58% of people with Type 1 diabetes, and 64% of people with Type 2 diabetes had cholesterol levels above 5mmol/l (27). However, at the same time, the number of people with cholesterol levels above 5mmol/l in the general population was significantly higher, with most groups of men and women above 55 years old having around 80-90% of people with cholesterol levels above 5mmol/l (3). In this instance it is important to specifically look at cholesterol levels in people aged 55 years and above, since it is around this age that the incidence of diabetes rapidly increases (28).

It is interesting that most risk factors associated with cardiovascular disease have a higher prevalence in people with diabetes. For example, 47% of women who have diabetes have high blood pressure, compared with just 15% of women having high blood pressure in the general population. A similar trend is found with the number of people who are above their ideal body weight (28). However, when it comes to cholesterol, diabetes is associated with lower levels. This may even suggest that having a higher cholesterol level is somehow protective against diabetes. Or put another way: low cholesterol increases the risk of having diabetes.

Summary

We are told that the average cholesterol level in the UK is too high. However, by comparing cholesterol levels with other countries around the World: the average level for the UK is low for Europe and similar to World averages.

If cholesterol really is such an important risk factor, then surely we would see at least some correlation with the data from various countries. There are not many examples that support the cholesterol idea, and there are many more examples that contradict it.

There is significant evidence to show that the rate of heart disease actually increases in most age groups when cholesterol levels are reduced. Cholesterol is a vital substance that is needed throughout the whole body. Reducing cholesterol levels to some theoretical value is an experiment never attempted before in history and the effects may be extremely detrimental to health.

A huge amount of money has been spent on 'educating' the general public about the 'dangers' of cholesterol but the alleged risks associated with cholesterol are not supported by the available evidence.

CHAPTER 8

Medicate the Masses!

*"A lie gets halfway around the world before the truth has
a chance to get its pants on."*
Sir Winston Leonard Spenser Churchill

By far, the most widely prescribed medications used to alter cholesterol levels are a group of drugs known as *statins*. There are a number of different statins, with different brand names, for example: *Atorvastatin (Lipitor, Torvast)*, *Fluvastatin (Lescol)*, *Pravastatin (Pravachol)*, *Rosuvastatin*, and *Simvastatin (Zocor, Lipex)*. The companies that make these drugs include: Merck, AstraZeneca, Bristol-Myers Squibb and Pfizer.

Any benefit associated with statins is said to be primarily due to their action of lowering LDLs (so called 'bad' cholesterol) and at the same time slightly increasing HDLs (so called 'good' cholesterol) within the body. The action of statins also has the effect of lowering the total cholesterol level. Statins achieve this by blocking the production of cholesterol in the liver.

The production of cholesterol in the liver involves a complex sequence of biochemical reactions. At each stage in this process, specific enzymes (biochemicals) are needed in order to progress to the next stage. Statins block the action of an enzyme used early on in this sequence.

The technical name for a statin drug is a *HMG-CoA Reductase Inhibitor* because it inhibits the enzyme *HMG-CoA Reductase*. Blocking this enzyme has the effect of preventing all downstream biochemical reactions that would normally continue after this point. Hence the manufacture of cholesterol in the liver is prevented. This is illustrated in figure 8A. Since most of the body's cholesterol is made in the liver, this has the effect of significantly lowering blood cholesterol levels.

The action that statins have on the production of cholesterol in the liver is similar to a factory manufacturing motor cars that does not have an operator to assemble the wheels of the car. Of course, a motor car cannot be manufactured without wheels, so its production will stop at the point in the production line at which the operator would normally assemble the wheels – in the same way, cholesterol cannot be manufactured without a specific enzyme being available, and its production in the liver will stop at the point when this enzyme is needed.

According to Dr Malcolm Kendrick, scientists have tried to use drugs to block cholesterol synthesis at various other stages in the sequence associated with its production, however the results were disastrous. Drugs that acted elsewhere in cholesterol synthesis resulted in problems such as "death of the surrounding organism" (1).

The sequence of biochemical steps shown in figure 8A is not used solely for the production of cholesterol. This sequence is also necessary for the production of a wide range of other molecules as well. Therefore, blocking the production of the cholesterol molecule also has the effect of blocking a large number of other substances.

Going back to our motor car analogy; imagine that this factory produces not only cars, but also motor cycles, lorries and buses. If the operator who assembles the wheels is not available, then not just the cars, but all of these vehicles are prevented from being manufactured.

The fact that statins prevent the production of other molecules within the body has a number of implications. For example, one of the many substances that are blocked by statins is a compound called *Coenzyme Q10 (CoQ10)*. This is a naturally occurring compound found in every cell of the body. CoQ10 is sometimes referred to as *ubiquinone*, which comes from the word *ubiquitous*, meaning 'found everywhere'. CoQ10 is vitally important for the production of energy at the cellular level. This energy is required for all muscles to function. The heart is of course a muscle and it cannot function if there is a deficiency of CoQ10.

A deficiency of CoQ10 can contribute to heart failure. Heart failure is the term used when the heart becomes less efficient at pumping blood around the body. Therefore, one potential effect of statins is that they may actually cause heart problems, even though they are designed to prevent them.

A study published in the *Archives of Neurology,* concluded that even brief exposure to a statin drug (in this case atorvastatin for 30 days) "causes a marked decrease in blood CoQ10 concentration", and "widespread inhibition of CoQ10 synthesis could explain the most commonly reported adverse effects of statins" (2).

Another study concluded that side effects related to statins, including *cardiomyopathy* (a serious disease in which the heart muscle becomes inflamed and does not work as well as it should) "are far more common than previously published" (3). This study found that these effects were reversible by stopping the statin drug and adding a supplement of CoQ10.

It is difficult to obtain reliable statistics on the incidence of heart failure. The situation may be influenced by an aging population, and there may be many more actual cases of heart failure than are being reported (4). However, this condition is increasing in countries that prescribe statins. In the UK, the British Heart Foundation suggested in the year 2002 that hospital admissions for heart failure are set to increase 50% during the next 25 years (5). In the United States, where 13 million people take a statin, hospitalisations for heart failure in 2004 were almost three times what they were in 1979: rising from 402,000 to 1,101,000 (6).

Patients with signs of heart failure are routinely excluded from statin drug trials (7, 8). Therefore, it is very difficult to establish if indeed there is a link between statins and heart failure. If heart failure is not listed as a potential side effect, then doctors may not make the association and may assume that heart failure is simply part of the patient's general condition.

A number of other studies provide further evidence that statins reduce CoQ10 levels (9 - 11). The authors of these studies highlight a concern about the wider range of potential side effects associated with this. This is discussed in more detail in chapter 10.

The pharmaceutical industry and some doctors have been very busy converting huge numbers of healthy people into patients. Between the years 1986 and 2005 the number of prescriptions given in the UK for statin drugs increased by 14, 300% (12). In 2007, the number of people in the UK taking these drugs was reported to be between 3 million (13) and 3.4 million (14).

In 2006, the National Institute for Health and Clinical Excellence (NICE) issued new recommendations for the use of statins. This report recommended that statins should be used for anyone who

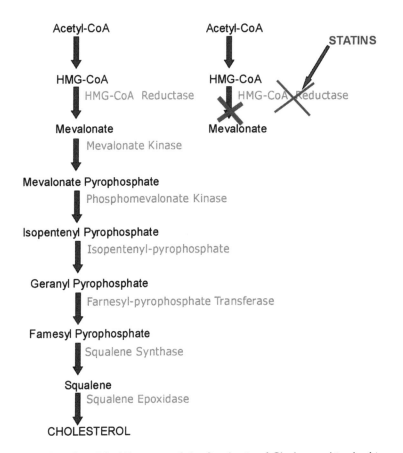

Figure 8A. Simplified Diagram of the Synthesis of Cholesterol in the Liver Showing How Statins Block HMG-CoA Reductase.

has a 20% or greater risk of developing cardiovascular disease over the next 10 years (15). This meant that up to 5.2 million people, in England alone, suddenly became 'eligible' for statin use (16).

In 2008, the UK government announced that everyone between the ages of 40 and 74 in England will be given a health check for heart disease. Professor Boyle, the government's national director for heart disease in England, has stated that this may more than double the number of people taking statins in the UK, and may increase the number to as many as 7 million people (17, 18).

When a person is put on to a statin drug they are instructed to take it everyday for the rest of their life. The British Heart Foundation states that the body does not stop making cholesterol and cholesterol levels will rise if the medication is discontinued – therefore it is necessary to keep taking the statin indefinitely (19).

Let us take a step back and think about this for a second. We are being told that in the UK there are millions of people who have a disease that is so serious that they require medication everyday for the rest of their lives. Along with this they will also need regular check-ups with their doctor in order to monitor the effects of the drugs.

This suggests that all of these people have a condition where their body is making too much cholesterol. If their cholesterol levels are too high, what is the cause of this? Is it due to a genetic fault? It seems extremely unlikely that millions of people have faulty genes causing high cholesterol levels.

There are some conditions that are known to increase cholesterol levels: such as in the case of a low thyroid function. The thyroid gland is one of the main hormone producing glands within the body. It plays an important role in many life supporting functions and controls our metabolic rate. It has been known for decades that low thyroid function (medically known as *hypothyroidism*) can increase cholesterol levels. A number of experts have the opinion that hypothyroidism is more common than is currently reported, but again, it is unlikely to account for the majority of the suggested cases of 'high' cholesterol.

It is also important to keep in mind that the number of people with suggested 'high' cholesterol is much greater than the millions who are eligible for statin use. For example, around 80% of people aged 45 to 64 have a cholesterol level above the suggested target of 5mmol/l (20).

It would seem logical to suggest that if some people do have a 'high' cholesterol level (assuming that this is indeed high rather than just being normal for them as an individual) then this has to be due to something associated with their lifestyle habits. Eventually we may understand the interaction between lifestyle and cholesterol levels, but the information that we are being *fed* at the moment does not fit the available evidence.

The proposed cause of having high cholesterol (eating too much saturated fat), as we have seen in chapters 5 and 6, is false and has never been proven. To the point where the cholesterol proponents themselves now state that diet does not affect cholesterol levels significantly. So what is causing so many people to have this suggested high level of cholesterol that requires 'life saving' statins?

The organisations that are promoting the almost indiscriminate use of statins do not seem interested in answering this question. Perhaps this is because most people who are prescribed statins do not need them? After all, the suggested condition of having 'high cholesterol' is in fact a normal level of cholesterol for the vast majority of people in the UK As we have seen from chapter 7, average cholesterol levels in the UK have not increased, but have decreased slightly. In addition, cholesterol levels in the UK are very close to the global average, and lower than average for Europe. Perhaps the cholesterol problem does not exist, but is merely a convenient idea being used to convince more people to take expensive statin drugs?

Statins are being increasingly prescribed to people who consider themselves to be fit and well. We are told that this is done in an attempt to prevent people from having their first heart attack. In medical terminology this is called *primary prevention*. However, it is very well established that 99% of people who take statins for primary prevention, do not benefit from the drugs at all. Even the strongest supporters of statins admit this (17, 18).

It also seems absurd that the British Heart Foundation can offer no other advice to reduce cholesterol levels than to continue to take statin drugs. If the suggested cholesterol problem really does exist, there must be a cause, and addressing this cause would relieve the problem. Of course, finding the cause of a fictitious problem is much more difficult.

The threshold by which people became 'eligible' for statin use was also lowered in the United States, leading to millions more people being put on satins. This raised questions when it was revealed that eight out of nine of the experts involved had links to the pharmaceutical companies that make statins (21).

Some people may indeed have a higher than average cholesterol level. This may or may not indicate a problem for them as an individual. It may be a sign of a bad lifestyle or it may be normal for them. As we have seen in chapter 5, cholesterol levels in people simply follow a normal distribution. In addition: more people die of heart disease with low cholesterol than with high cholesterol, most people who have a heart attack have an average cholesterol level, and high cholesterol is associated with a longer life in some age groups. Therefore, when we consider the population as a whole, the wide spread use of statins could actually be causing more problems than it is solving.

There are studies showing that statins do reduce the risk of heart disease in some people. However in most of these studies, lives have not been saved because the people taking the statins have died more frequently of other causes. In the small number of studies that have shown statins to provide a reduction in deaths from all causes, the benefits have been very small and over-stated by the authors. In addition, there are frequent, and sometimes very serious, side effects associated with statins - this raises important questions about their use. We shall also see in chapter 11 that any benefit provided by statins is due to mechanisms that have nothing to do with cholesterol at all.

To make matters even worse the use of statin drugs has been extended to groups of people for which the drugs have either not been adequately tested on, or have actually been shown to have a detrimental effect.

People who do not benefit from statins include all women and the elderly. Dr John Abramson from Harvard Medical School and Dr James Wright from the University of British Columbia, published a study in the *Lancet* in January 2007 (22). This study stated that there was no evidence to show giving statins to women of any age protected them from heart disease. It also showed that statins did not provide any benefit for the 3,239 men and women above 69 years of age who were studied.

Dr Malcolm Kendrick, a GP who has worked with the European Society of Cardiology, said in response to this study: "I hope this at least makes people question things and then maybe the truth will come out that we are having the wool pulled over our eyes. There is no reason for women to take statins" (23).

Actually, the lack of any benefits in the use of statins for women has been reported in the scientific literature for some time. In 2004 an analysis was published in the *Journal of the American Medical Association*. This article synthesised all studies between 1966 and 2003 in order to investigate the effect of using drugs to lower cholesterol in women (24). The authors concluded that lowering cholesterol levels with drugs did not reduce the number of deaths from all causes. For women who already had cardiovascular disease, lowering cholesterol levels reduced the risk of having a heart attack, but even in this very high risk group the death rate was not reduced.

Even back in 1992, there was a review published in the *Lancet* to show that observations about heart disease found in men cannot be assumed to be the same for women (25). In this study the authors found that women in the highest cholesterol group (above 7.2 mmol/l) had lower heart disease death rates than men in the lowest cholesterol group (less than 5.0 mmol/l).

It seems strange then, that the British Heart Foundation states that "The evidence that we have so far indicates that statins are equally effective in both sexes" (19). We should all ask them and any doctor who puts women on statins, where their evidence is in support of this? – the response is likely to be just an embarrassed look.

Another study published in *The New England Journal of Medicine*, included 5011 patients who were 60 years of age or above. These people were spit into two groups: one group was given a statin drug and the other was given a placebo. When the two groups were compared, the group who were given the statin drug had a much lower level of so called 'bad' cholesterol (LDLs). In fact the level of LDLs in this group was about half the level in the group given the placebo. However, there were no benefits provided or lives saved as a result of this (26).

In April 2008, a BBC Radio 4 program questioned the use of statins in the elderly (18). During the program, a doctor from Manchester in the UK described how he had asked the National Health Service (NHS) for any evidence they have that statins are beneficial for the elderly. Out of all the scientific literature that has been published in the western world, the NHS was not able to provide any such evidence.

Later in the same radio program (18), another doctor admitted that he prescribes statins to the elderly even though he does not have any evidence that they are beneficial. What is more worrying is the fact that this same doctor admitted that 80% of the work he does for patients is not evidence based. Patients and the general public assume, when a doctor gives advice or prescribes medication that these actions are based on scientific evidence that is obtained using a rigorous scientific process. As more people start to ask searching questions, it is increasingly revealed that a large proportion of medical practice is not evidence based at all.

The British Heart Foundation, in their informative booklet *Medicines for the Heart* fails to mention that statins are of no benefit to the elderly. It merely states that; "Statins are not suitable for people who have liver disease or who are pregnant or breastfeeding" (27).

Some experts are so enthusiastic about the use of statins that they are advocating their use for even more people. Not content with the 5.2 million just in England alone who can be prescribed statins, they have suggested that millions more people are available for *statination*. For example, authors of the Heart Protection Study Collaborative claimed that people as young as 35 years with a 1% chance of heart disease or stroke would benefit from a lifetime use of statins (28).

Much more worrying is the fact that some 'experts' are proposing to put children as young as eight years onto statins (29). This was suggested by the American Academy of Pediatrics (AAP) in July 2008. The academy has stated that the benefit of giving statins at a younger age outweighs the risks associated with the drugs (30). This viewpoint can not be substantiated, since there is absolutely no evidence that statins are effective or safe for children. The academy is extrapolating the risks and benefits that have been observed in adults and assuming the same is true for young children.

Even if we do base our assessment of this issue on the data available from studies done on adults, it is clear that the benefits do not outweigh the risks (as we have seen throughout this book). Cholesterol is essential for proper growth and development. It would be nothing short of a criminal offense to routinely screen children for eligibility for cholesterol lowering drugs. It is difficult to decide which is more frightening: the prospect of children routinely being given statins or the fact that an organisation such as the AAP think that this is appropriate.

Another worrying state of affairs is that statins are also now available over the counter without a prescription, in the form of *Zocor Heart-Pro*.

Cost / Profit Associated With Statins

Whilst many researchers have doubts about the proposed benefits of statins and the level of safety associated with them, others have questioned their cost-effectiveness. Statins are expensive and place a significant burden on the resources of the health care system in the UK, representing the single greatest drug expenditure by the National Health Service (NHS). When the entire cost of treatment is taken into account it is estimated that the NHS may be spending as much as £2 billion each year on statins (31, 32).

In 2008, the NHS is celebrating its sixty year anniversary. Value for money in the NHS has been placed under scrutiny since funding has risen substantially. People should be made aware that billions of pounds are being wasted on medications that have minuscule benefit for the majority of people who take them.

The amount of money being spent on statins in the UK represents approximately £41 per person of the adult population per year. This money could be invested into any number of more worthwhile areas of health care or could even be used to build two and a half Wembley Stadiums.

Statins are the biggest selling prescription drugs of all time. They generate more money for the pharmaceutical companies than any other form of medication, with global sales of US$26 billion in 2004 (21) and almost US$28 billion in 2006 (33).

One of the statins, with the brand name Lipitor, generated almost US$13 billion in revenue for its manufacturer, Pfizer in 2006. This is an unprecedented amount of revenue for drug companies. The other top selling drugs on Pfizer's company accounts generate nowhere near this amount, with sales ranging from just US$1 billion to US$4 billion (34).

Millions of people around the world are taking statins to reduce their cholesterol levels. For example, there were more than 76 million prescriptions issued for statins in the United States in the year 2000 (35). Despite this intensive prescription of statins, reports suggest that they have not made any difference to the incidence of heart disease. An article published in the *Journal of the American College of Cardiology* in 2006, showed that there was no change in the risk of developing heart disease between the years 1988 and 2002 (36).

'Unexpected' Results

Not content with the use of statins, the pharmaceutical companies have been trying to introduce drugs that have more specific effects on cholesterol. For example, drugs have been tested that specifically target HDL 'cholesterol' (so called 'good' cholesterol). In November 2007, an article was published in the *New England Journal of Medicine* detailing a trial used to test the effects of using a drug to increase HDL 'cholesterol' along with a statin to reduce LDL 'cholesterol' (37). This trial was terminated prematurely because of a significant increase in deaths and heart attacks in people who took both medications.

The drugs achieved a 72% increase in HDLs and a 25% decrease in LDLs. According to supporters of the cholesterol idea this is a very favourable change in the cholesterol profile, however despite this, there was a 40% increase in deaths from cardiovascular causes. Deaths from other causes were also increased - by a factor of two. It is not clear if the increased number of deaths were due to the drug itself or the supposed 'favourable' changes in cholesterol. However, it does raise serious questions about the idea of increasing 'good' cholesterol through medication (38).

This example provides us with a better appreciation of the financial aspects associated with cholesterol drugs and the interests that the pharmaceutical industry has vested in them. As a result of the disappointing outcome of this trial, the manufacturer (Pfizer) announced that it was halting all clinical testing of this new drug. Consequently, the company's market value fell by US$21 billion overnight and ten thousand people had to lose their job (39).

Why Do Doctors Agree With the Cholesterol Idea?

By now the reader may be asking: if the cholesterol idea is wrong, why do so many doctors believe it? Or: if there are big concerns about the use of statins, why do so many doctors prescribe them? These are very good questions and in order to answer them we need to consider the complex world that doctors are forced to work in, and some of the changes that have taken place in how medical research is conducted. These issues are discussed in the next chapter. For many readers this will provide a shocking insight into some of the limitations of contemporary medicine and medical research.

It is also important to realise that not all doctors do agree with the cholesterol idea. Ever since cholesterol was first suggested as the villain in heart disease, there have been a large number of doctors and researchers who have challenged the hypothesis.

In the immediate future, the prescription of statins is set to increase. Many people will feel that they do not want to accept these drugs but may not have the confidence to fully question their doctor about them. The resources for this book at www.29billion.com include a standard letter that can be used by readers to probe their doctor on this issue.

CHAPTER 9

How Did We Get Here?

If the cholesterol idea is wrong and is not based on scientific evidence, it is logical to question why so many people, including a large number of doctors, have been taken in by it. This question can be answered through an appreciation of the general environment that doctors now work in.

Many readers will be surprised to learn that there are a number of significant problems with medical journals and the way medical research is published. Few people, apart from medical researchers themselves, have the time or the inclination to investigate these problems. However, they certainly do exist, and they affect whether or not a drug is considered effective and safe.

It will not however be a surprise to most people that medicine is generally influenced far too much by drug companies. But there is significant evidence that this problem is getting out of control. Inappropriate connections between researchers/doctors and the pharmaceutical industry are hindering the scientific process and affect government policy.

Many doctors are extremely uncomfortable with the current situation, but their voices seldom reach the general public. The aim of this chapter is to highlight just a few of the problems faced by the medical community. This will help readers to appreciate how the cholesterol idea could have been so widely accepted in the absence of sufficient scientific evidence to support it.

The Business of Selling Drugs

Pharmaceutical companies are of course a business just like any other, and the people who work for them want to increase profitability. Shareholders also want to see a return on their investment. It is only natural that these companies want to sell more drugs and there is evidence that they have been very successful in doing this.

For example, in the UK, the Office for National Statistics publishes data concerning the number of prescriptions written in England between 1996 and 2006. During this ten year period there was an increase in the number of prescription items from 485 million to 752 million per year. The number of prescriptions per person in the population increased from 10 to 14.8. In fact the number of prescription items has increased significantly every year for the last ten years (1).

Some may argue that this is a good thing and an indication that new drugs are being made available to patients. In some cases this may be true; however, overall the trend may be more worrying.

Richard Smith worked for the *British Medical Journal (BMJ)* for 25 years and was Editor and Chief Executive of the BMJ Publishing Group from 1991 to 2004. During this time he became one of the most influential people within medicine. In his book titled *The Trouble with Medical Journals* (2), which is published by The Royal Society of Medicine, he analyses the problems and current trends in medical publishing. The book provides a fascinating and highly readable account of these issues. It is highly recommended to anyone (including those without a scientific background) who wishes to gain an insight into the world of medical research and how it influences our daily lives.

Richard Smith does not examine the subject of cholesterol, but he does explain how the pharmaceutical companies, although powerful and influential, are experiencing a "productivity crisis" (2). In order for these companies to grow and increase profits they need to develop innovative drugs that genuinely provide significant benefits for patients. Unfortunately the number of pharmacological breakthroughs in this respect have been much fewer than was hoped for (2).

It was hoped that new drugs would be discovered for the ever increasing degenerative diseases suffered by huge numbers of people in the developed world. However, these attempts have been unsuccessful. The number of new drugs approved in the United States by the Food and Drug Administration (FDA) in 2002 was significantly less than in previous years (2). Pharmaceutical companies have been forced to look at other ways to achieve business growth. This includes increasing marketing efforts to get more people to use their drugs, and creating new diseases: or converting more people into patients.

Some authors describe these activities as "disease mongering" (3, 4). They are concerned about the "invisible and unregulated attempts to change public perceptions about health and illness in order to widen markets for new drugs" (3).

Barbara Mintzes, in an article published in the *Public Library of Science (PLoS) Medicine* (4), describes the various forms that disease mongering by pharmaceutical companies can take. This includes:

- Promotion of anxiety about future ill-health in healthy people
- Exaggerating the number of people affected by the 'disease'

- Promotion of aggressive drug treatment for mild symptoms
- Introducing new conditions that are hard to distinguish from normal life, such as social anxiety disorder
- Promoting drugs as the first solution for problems previously not considered medical, such as: disruptive classroom behaviour or problematic sexual relationships

An advert was placed in a London newspaper in February 2008 designed to recruit people to take part in a drug trial. The trial is for a condition called *Hypoactive Sexual Desire Disorder (HSDD)*, otherwise known as: a low sex drive. Giving this problem a long technical name and publicising it creates a new disease or condition that requires new drugs to treat it. Traditionally, this kind of problem has been dealt with in other ways, without medication.

A lot of money can be made from healthy people who believe they are sick (3), since disease mongering exploits our deepest fears of suffering and death (5). Substantial and lucrative professional careers have been built on the pursuit of new diseases or risk factors for disease (5). The pharmaceutical companies are exploiting opportunities in this area for business growth by making more people aware of certain 'conditions'.

In some cases more emphasis appears to be placed on risk factors than on the disease itself. High cholesterol has become synonymous with heart disease to the extent that the management of cholesterol levels has become more of a concern than the prevention of heart disease.

A number of studies have been completed that focus solely on cholesterol levels. One study looked at how many people in

England have low HDL levels (so called 'good' cholesterol) and how many people are taking cholesterol lowering drugs (6). Another study looked at HDL levels in various European countries (7). According to the supporters of the cholesterol idea, low HDL levels contribute to the risk for developing heart disease. Therefore, investigations such as these may seem valid, but they create an impression that having the suggested 'risk factor' is the same as having the disease.

The authors use the data obtained to conclude that more people need to take cholesterol lowering drugs, or additional drugs should be used that specifically target HDLs. This conclusion is reached without regard to the many factors that contribute to heart disease.

By just looking at one of the suggested risk factors we lose sight of the main objective: which is to actually save lives. In the previous chapter we discussed a clinical trial for a drug used specifically to increase HDL levels. Readers will recall that this trial was terminated because of an increase in deaths and heart attacks in people who took this drug along with a statin. This is what can happen when focus is placed solely on risk factors, especially in a condition such as heart disease that has numerous complex mechanisms associated with it.

Drug companies have been restructuring their organisations: shifting more of their resources into marketing and 'education' so that they can take full advantage of the opportunities. In American research-based drug companies, the number of people employed in research and development has fallen 2% since 1995, but marketing staff have increased by 59%. Twice as many people are now employed in marketing than in research and development (2). It has been estimated that around US$10,000 a year is spent on marketing to each doctor in the United States and that around US$2.5 billion was spent in 2000 on marketing to consumers (2).

The pharmaceutical industry spends millions of dollars supporting the 'education' of doctors. It has been estimated that 99% of doctors use information provided by pharmaceutical companies in their clinical practice (5). If the prescribing of drugs and profits for drug companies were not affected by this support, it would not be offered (5).

Doctors and Drug Companies

Pharmaceutical companies should be allowed to sell their products to doctors. This is a necessary part of the overall process involved in medicine. However, connections between doctors and drug companies can in many ways become inappropriate and have an unnatural influence on prescription habits. This is particularly true when doctors who hold influential positions determining treatment protocols are supported by the pharmaceutical companies. Readers will recall from chapter 8 that the panel of expects responsible for deciding who should be prescribed statins, was mostly made up of doctors who were supported by statin manufacturers. Eight out of nine of the experts had connections with the companies that make the drugs. No surprise then that the threshold for statin use was lowered: making millions more people eligible to use the drugs and massively increasing the size of the market for them.

According to a survey completed in America, 94% of doctors have some kind of link with the pharmaceutical industry (8). The frequency of different types of connections is listed below:

- Receiving food and drinks in the workplace – 83%
- Receiving drug samples from a sales representative – 78%
- Reimbursement for costs associated with professional meetings – 35%

Other payments are received for consulting, serving as a speaker, serving on an advisory board, and enrolling patients on clinical trials (8, 9).

Some doctors are of the opinion that these ties with industry do not influence the prescribing of drugs. However, there are certain social obligations associated with gifts and human beings often feel the need to reciprocate in some way when they receive one – even if the gift was something that they didn't want. Likewise, if a doctor has received excellent hospitality from a pharmaceutical company during a seminar or conference, they are less likely to be openly critical of the company's drugs. Doctors are of course only human like the rest of us.

Interestingly, a survey conducted on medical students found that 86% thought it was improper for a politician to receive a gift, but only 46% thought it was improper for themselves to receive a gift of a similar value from a pharmaceutical company (10).

Some positive outcomes have been found as a result of these links with drug companies, such as doctors being better able to identify the treatment for complicated illnesses (10). However, most studies have found negative outcomes, such as:

- Doctors not being able to identify wrong claims about medication
- Doctors requesting new, more expensive drugs that have no demonstrated benefit over existing ones

- Increased prescription rates
- Irrational prescribing behaviour (10)

Prescription rates and practices are probably compounded by short consultation times with doctors. A study published in the *British Medical Journal* in 2002, compared average consultation times in six European countries. The average consultation time with doctors in the UK was 9.4 minutes. However the authors of the study highlighted the fact that in reality, average consultation times may be lower, since the doctors in their study had lower workloads than the average for the country as a whole. The consultations in the study were also videotaped: which may have influenced the consultation time. Interestingly, in Belgium and Switzerland, where patients pay the doctor directly at the end of their consultation, the average consultation time was 15 minutes and 15.6 minutes respectively (11).

Bias in Publishing Results

Clinical drug trials are increasingly sponsored by the pharmaceutical industry. Various studies have found that when a pharmaceutical company sponsors research into a drug, the results are considerably more likely to show the drug in a favourable light. Systematic bias occurs when the drugs being tested are made by the company funding the research (12).

In addition, drug trials that show favourable results are more likely to be published (13), and pharmaceutical companies have attempted to prevent studies that show unfavourable results (for their products) from being published (12).

An example of this can be found in the *ENHANCE* trial. This was a two year trial to test the effects of using a drug called *ezetimibe* in conjunction with a statin to achieve greater reductions in cholesterol. The people who took part in the trial were split into two groups: one group was given ezetimibe and the statin, and the other group were given just the statin. LDL levels (so called 'bad' cholesterol) were reduced to a considerably lower level in the group who were given both ezetimibe and the statin (14). According to the cholesterol idea, these greater reductions in LDL levels should result in greater reductions in heart disease compared with the people who just took the statin. The greater reductions in LDLs should also reduce the build up of plaque within arteries. However, the researchers found the opposite to be true. Rather than providing any benefit, the addition of ezetimibe actually lead to a slight increase in the amount of plaque found in the main arteries that supply blood and oxygen to the brain (15).

The results of the ENHANCE trial raises questions about the idea that cholesterol levels are related to the build up of plaque in arteries. But this issue is over-shadowed by the fact that the drug companies attempted to hide these results from the public for as long as possible.

The ENHANCE trial ended in April 2006, but the companies that make the drug being tested; Merck and Schering-Plough, did not report the results until January 2008. Even then, the results were only released after pressure from Congress in America (14), and after articles started to appear in the news media questioning the delay (14, 16).

The companies blamed the complexity of the data for the delay. A spokesman for Schering said the delay was unrelated to the negative findings and that the results were not known until two weeks before they were released. However, deadlines were repeatedly missed for reporting the results and in the meantime, millions of people continued to take the drug unaware of the negative results of the trial (14). Global sales of the drug in question were US$5 billion in 2007 (17). In England alone, more than two million prescriptions were written in the two years prior to the release of the results, costing the National Health Service £74 million (17).

All of this is bad enough, but there were also problems with the registration of the ENHANCE trial. An official register of clinical trials is used to stop researchers changing the objective of the trial that is being conducted. Since these changes could be done in order to cover-up unfavourable results. The ENHANCE trial was not registered until 18 months after the trial had ended and the objective of the trial has been reported to have been altered in the register (18).

Subsequent studies have been completed on ezetimibe showing that the use of this drug in conjunction with a statin increases the risk for cancer (19). Investigators dismissed this as a chance finding (20), but significant questions remain (21). Patients are being expected to continue to take this drug on faith, potentially exposing themselves to serious side effects. The drug is used under the trade names *Zetia*, *Vytorin*, *Ezetrol*, and *Inegy*.

The ENHANCE trial is just one example of problems that can arise when focus is placed on suggested risk factors rather than on the disease itself. In order for drugs to be approved by the FDA in America, it is not necessary to show benefits in terms of a reduction in heart disease risk – merely demonstrating that the drug lowers 'bad' cholesterol (LDLs) is enough to get it approved (22). This is a dangerous and risky approach for patients, and it distracts research away from finding the true causes of a disease.

In the ENHANCE trial the suggested risk factor (in this case cholesterol) was significantly reduced, but this resulted in absolutely no benefit for patients. Even if the trial was designed to investigate a valid hypothesis, the results should have been released immediately. As stated by Ben Goldacre, writing in the *Guardian* newspaper "the data belongs to patients – and to the people whose bodies are used" (18).

Delaying the results of a trial, or never publishing the results, is one way that publication bias is introduced. Another way is publishing studies more than once. Researchers often perform what is termed a *systematic review* of all studies that have been completed on a drug in order to gain an overall view on the effectiveness of treatment. If positive results are published more than once and negative results not published at all, the conclusions of a systematic review will be affected substantially. The end result may be that patients are given toxic and expensive treatments that do not benefit them (2).

A paper published in the *New England Journal of Medicine* investigated the extent of publication bias in antidepressant drug trials. It was found that 31% of the trials had not been published and that almost all of the unpublished trials showed negative results associated with the drug being tested. According to the published studies 94% of trials found favourable results for the drug, but when the unpublished trials are included only 51% of the trials had a favourable result (23).

In February 2008, Professor Irving Kirsch and colleagues conducted a detailed analysis of all the clinical trial data submitted to the FDA on antidepressant drugs (24). They analysed all of the data: both published and unpublished. The conclusion they reached was that antidepressant drugs were no more effective than a *placebo*. This caused an outcry, since the drugs are used by 40 million people worldwide (25). It may be true that some people have benefited from taking antidepressant drugs but the benefits appear to be due to the *placebo effect*. This example shows just how the effectiveness of drugs can be exaggerated if data about them is not published. This publication bias can help pharmaceutical companies to make more profit.

News Media

Most people do not see their doctor regularly, and as we have seen, consultation times are often short in duration. Therefore the media represents the most significant source of health information for the general public.

Television, radio and newspaper medical reporters have a difficult job. They must be accurate, authoritative, and compassionate. They also need to understand the terminology, physiology, epidemiology, study design, and statistical analysis to keep health news in context for the viewer/listener/reader (26).

The way information about drugs is presented through the media has a huge impact on the share price of pharmaceutical companies. In February 2008, Jean-Pierre Garnier, chief executive of the drugs giant GlaxoSmithKline (GSK), gave a presentation in London in which he discussed the reasons for the disappointing financial results for the company during the previous year. The financial results were poor because of reports about the company's diabetes drug *Avandia* being linked with heart problems. Garnier partly blamed the media for the drop in sales that resulted from this (27).

The negative reports about Avandia came after a study published in the *New England Journal of Medicine* found that the drug was associated with an increased risk for having a heart attack (28). The author of the study was Dr Steven Nissen, a cardiologist at the respected Cleveland Clinic. The study was particularly important because heart disease is the most serious complication associated with diabetes. As a result of this published paper and the media reports communicating it to the general public, more than US$10 billion was wiped off the value of GSK during afternoon trading in the United States (29).

At the time, GSK strongly disagreed with the study published by Dr Nissen and said that the conclusions reached were based on incomplete evidence (30). However, Dr Nissen was also part of the scientific team that completed an analysis of the available data on the drug *Vioxx*. This analysis found that Vioxx increased heart attack and stroke risks. A patient trial was subsequently completed that came to the same conclusion. This forced Vioxx to be withdrawn (31).

The debate about the increased risk of suffering a heart attack while taking Avandia has continued. This is another example where people are being expected to carry on taking a drug on faith. One study, supported by GSK, stated that the data was insufficient (32). However, the same study did find evidence of a significant increase in the risk of *heart failure* with Avandia (32). GSK announced that it would make chances to the labeling of the drug in Europe to inform people about this risk (33).

A large clinical trial started in 2001 (the *ACCORD* trial) that included a range of diabetes drugs, including Avandia (34). This trial was designed to evaluate the use of drugs to intensively lower blood glucose levels compared with the use of drugs to moderately lower blood glucose. The trial was due to be completed in 2009, however, the use of drugs to intensively lower blood glucose was stopped 17 months early because of an increased number of deaths in this group.

Since the ACCORD trial included a range of drugs, it is not possible to determine which drugs caused the increased deaths. GSK have pointed out that there is no direct link between Avandia and the increased deaths found during the trial (35). However, Avandia was used more extensively in the group that experienced more deaths.

Avandia may or may not increase the risk of having a heart attack and/or increase the risk of death, but this case provides an example of the media just doing its job – informing patients of the potential risks associated with a widely used drug. Media reports such as this may not be good for share holders' profits but they are absolutely vital to patients. Even a small increase in risk in a fragile population of patients with diabetes is of considerable concern (36).

However, journalists can unwittingly become 'mouthpieces' for those with vested interests (26). Pharmaceutical companies can use the media to portray exaggerated benefits associated with their drugs. This is what happened in the case of the follow up of the *West of Scotland Coronary Prevention Study (WOSCOPS)* which appeared as a major success for statins in the media. A closer look at this study shows that some of the conclusions reached were misleading. This example is discussed in more detail in chapter 13.

Medical Journals: Powerful, but Also Problematic

The examples described above show how influential medical journals are. Most people think of medical journals as dull and obscure, however the content of them influences the lives of us all. Not only do they affect what doctors do with individual patients and the actions taken by public health authorities on whole populations, but they also influence how we think about birth, death, pain and sickness (2). However, there are a number of serious problems with medical journals.

Pharmaceutical companies generate influence through medical journals in a number of ways. One obvious way is through advertising. Advertising in journals can increase the prescribing of drugs (2). A large number of doctors receive journals such as the *British Medical Journal*, the *New England Journal of Medicine*, and the *Journal of the American Medical Association*, for free because of the financial support the journals get from pharmaceutical company advertising. Publishers of medical journals are always worried that these companies will cut back on advertising and they argue that advertising produces a better financial return for the pharmaceutical industry than employing more company representatives (2).

Authorship is also a serious problem with medical journals. Surprisingly the list of authors that appear at the top of a medical paper may not reflect true authorship. It has been stated that there are four types of lie: lies, damned lies, statistics, and the authorship lists of scientific papers (37). Scientific communities call this problem *ghost authorship*. Ghost authors are people who have contributed to a research study or been involved in writing the paper, but their name does not appear on the list of authors.

There are a number of implications associated with ghost authorship. One of the main concerns is that the ghost author is employed by a pharmaceutical company – this creates a conflict of interest that is not declared and may mean that the paper is not looked at in its true light. One study found that 75% of trials had ghost authors (38). In this case the ghost authors were statisticians who were employed by the pharmaceutical companies supporting the trials. Clinical trials are often complex and generate large datasets; the statistical report is a fundamental part of the research and has a crucial influence on what is written in the publication (38). Not declaring the statistician deceives the reader about the role of the supporting company.

Potential problems also exist with the *peer review* process. Richard Smith, in his book, explains these problems in detail: "Peer review is at the heart of all science – It is the method by which grants are allocated, papers published, academics promoted and Nobel prizes won. Yet it is hard to define ... and its defects are easier to identify than its attributes" (2).

Peer review could loosely be described as getting a third party to verify or make a decision about whether to publish a paper. Ideally the third party should not be connected with the research, have no competing interests, but still be in a position to technically appraise the methodology and findings. Richard Smith explains that peer review sometimes seems to be a simple case of someone saying "the paper looks all right to me" (2) and examples of a comprehensive, detailed review of a paper are difficult to find. These issues directly impact the quality of what gets published and what does not get published - influencing the conclusions that are reached about a wide range of medical conditions and treatment protocols.

Doctors Are Paid More If They Lower Your Cholesterol

In April 2004, the National Health Service (NHS) in the UK introduced the *Quality and Outcomes Framework (QOF)*. This is a kind of performance related pay and is applied to every general practitioner medical practice. QOF contains 146 quality indicators which doctors have to report on. The better the practice does in terms of these indicators, the more money it will get from the NHS.

Around half of the potential revenue from QOF is associated with indicators of clinical quality (39). Specific indicators have been identified for a range of common conditions. For example, a list of indicators has been identified for diabetes. These include body mass index (BMI) and blood glucose levels. The more diabetic patients that have a BMI and blood glucose level below a specified value, the more money the doctor will get from the NHS.

One of the problems with QOF is that many of the indicators are based on risk factors for disease and targets are set without regard to how they are achieved. There are performance measures, or targets, set for cholesterol.

If a patient has heart disease, diabetes or if they have had a stroke, doctors are expected to lower their cholesterol so that it is below 5mmol/l (millimoles per litre). If, say, 40% of a doctors diabetic patients have a cholesterol level below 5mmol/l, the doctor will be paid less than if 50% of diabetic patients have a cholesterol level below 5mmol/l. In summary, there is a strong financial incentive for doctors to lower the cholesterol levels of certain patients. Since the majority of people in the UK happen to naturally have a cholesterol level above 5mmol/l, the doctor has little choice but to put more people onto statins.

An article published in the *New England Journal of Medicine* describes the problems associated with performance measures being based on risk factors for disease (40). This paper cites a number of examples where the focus on the risk factor has actually caused more harm and increased the number of deaths.

CHAPTER 10

Safety of Statins

The reader will recall from previous chapters of this book that statins target so called 'bad' cholesterol (LDLs). Experts who are intent on describing HDLs and LDLs as 'good' and 'bad' respectively seem to be forgetting that these lipoproteins carry not just cholesterol, but other molecules around the body as well. For instance, HDLs and LDLs provide the main transport mechanism for a number of vital nutrients within the body. These include *coenzyme Q10 (CoQ10)*, *vitamin E*, and various *carotenoids* such as *beta-carotene* (1, 2).

Transportation of these vital nutrients via lipoproteins happens in a complex way. Interestingly the amount of cholesterol contained in a human lipoprotein is directly related to the quantity of vitamin E it contains. As cholesterol levels increase so do vitamin E levels. For some reason, in men, more vitamin E is carried in LDLs, however, in women more vitamin E is carried in HDLs (3). This provides further evidence that the way LDLs and HDLs work in the body is much more complicated than simply one of them being 'bad' and the other 'good'. In addition, do we know enough about the complex balance of lipoproteins in the body to alter them with drugs? Surely this can potentially cause problems with the transport of vital nutrients to tissues where they are needed.

The way that statins block the production of CoQ10 within the body has already been discussed in chapter 8. However, tissue levels of this vital substance are reduced even further when statins are used because of the reduction in the number of LDLs available to transport it to parts of the body where it is needed.

CoQ10, Vitamin E, beta-carotene and other carotenoids are antioxidants. Antioxidants are natural substances that exist as vitamins, minerals and other compounds. It is believed that these substances prevent the production of *free radicals*. Free radicals are unstable molecules that can attack healthy cells and lead to cancer or heart disease. Free radicals can also accelerate the aging process, cause complications with diabetes and contribute to a range of other disorders. The main process by which free radicals do damage is related to the normal action of *oxidation*: where molecules lose an *electron*. Antioxidants, such as the nutrients listed above serve as *electron donors* and deactivate the free radicals, preventing them from injuring cells.

Vitamin E, in addition to being an antioxidant, plays a number of other very important roles within the body. Some of these are listed below; taken from Robert Benowicz's book *Vitamins and You* (4):

Vitamin E:
- Ensures proper functioning of the circulatory system, the nervous system, digestive system, excretory system and the respiratory system
- Helps to maintain the integrity of cell membranes, including red blood cells, nerve cells, kidney tissues, the lungs and liver
- Promotes normal growth patterns and the body's ability to respond to stress
- Stimulates proper development and tone of the skeletal muscles, the heart and intestines (4).

Low blood levels of Vitamin E may be associated with a number of problems including disorders of the central nervous system, deterioration of the brain and progression of Alzheimer's disease. A low blood level of Vitamin E is also very predictive of heart disease – far more predictive than cholesterol or high blood pressure (5).

Statin manufacturers and their supporters would have us believe that side effects related to statins are rare and when they do occur are usually mild. They quote data from clinical trails showing a low rate of adverse reactions. Unfortunately the reality is very different. This is due, in part, to the fact that groups of people who are selected for clinical trials are chosen very carefully and are often very different from normal population groups.

Anthony Colpo in his book *The Great Cholesterol Con* (6) describes how researchers carefully screen for a wide range of people or existing medical conditions when recruiting participants for statin clinical trials. Colpo lists the exclusion criteria which includes: "women of childbearing age, those with a history of drug or alcohol abuse, poor mental function, heart failure, arrhythmia and other heart conditions, liver and kidney disorders, cancer, other serious diseases, and hypersensitivity to statins" (6). If any of the above applies to the person they are routinely excluded from the trial.

In addition to this, clinical trials often have a *run-in* period where even more people can be excluded. The participants will typically take the drug for a few weeks and if any adverse effects are experienced, or if the participant decides not to continue for any other reason, they are withdrawn from the trial. All of this means that the group who finally go into the actual trial are chosen precisely and are no longer representative of the general population.

An example of this can be seen in a recent trial conducted to evaluate a new drug aimed at increasing 'good' cholesterol. Of the 19,000 people assessed for eligibility, more than 2,000 were excluded before the run-in phase, and almost another 2,000 were excluded before the trial officially started (7). It may well be the case that some of these people were excluded for safety reasons, however the question remains about how many of the people excluded would ordinarily be prescribed statins in the real world.

In the United States, drugs are often approved on the basis that further clinical trials will be completed after the drug has been marketed (8). This post-marketing evaluation is critical, as highlighted in the case of *cerivastatin* (a cholesterol lowering statin drug) which was withdrawn from use in 2001 after it was linked to the deaths of 52 patients (9). It is estimated that more than ten percent of drugs after being approved, subsequently have to include one or more prominent *black-box* safety warning or are withdrawn from the market (8). A black-box safety warning is one that is added to the packaging of the drug and indicates that there may be very serious or life-threatening adverse effects associated with taking that drug. Despite the importance of post-marketing surveillance, in practice more than half of the studies promised by pharmaceutical companies are not started (10).

Many adverse effects are first recognised in the post-marketing surveillance process, and the frequency of side effects is likely to be understated because few doctors report them (11). The approval of a drug for clinical use "does not and cannot guarantee safety" (12). In addition, pharmaceutical companies may selectively publish only favourable results, leading to pharmaceutical industry bias (13) and a misrepresentation of the true situation.

Dr Malcolm Kendrick has written in the *British Medical Journal* about the potential adverse effects of statins (14). He explains that definite evidence comes from the US Food and Drug Administration adverse event reporting system - showing that between 1997 and 2004 one of the statin drugs (simvastatin) was reported as a direct cause of 49,350 adverse events and 416 deaths. Since adverse events are greatly under-reported, the actual figures are likely to be much higher (14).

Statins and Cancer

Statin manufacturers are very keen to quote clinical trials showing their drugs do not lead to an increased incidence of cancer. However most statin trials are just a few years in duration and cancer normally takes decades to develop. For example, smokers do not usually get cancer just a few years after taking up their first cigarette, but more often after a few decades of continuing with the habit. If statins do increase the risk of cancer, then this should be seen first in groups of people at high risk such as the elderly (11). The *PROSPER* trial has tested the effects of statins on older people (15), and it found that cancer diagnosis was more frequent for people who took the statin than those who did not. In this trial, that included people aged 70 to 82 years, any benefits that were achieved by slightly reducing the risk of heart disease were counteracted by the increased risk of cancer associated with the drug. This was seen even with just three years of follow-up. We do not know the longer-term implications for statins and cancer risk.

Another study published in the *Journal of the American College of Cardiology* stated in its conclusion that any cardiovascular benefits associated with low levels of LDL cholesterol may in part be offset by an increased risk of cancer (16).

Mental and Nervous System Problems

Cholesterol is vital for the development and function of the brain. It is therefore hardly surprising that mental and neurological complaints have been observed when cholesterol levels are reduced (11).

Duane Graveline is a former astronaut, aerospace medical research scientist, flight surgeon, family doctor and an author. One could assume that Dr Graveline is a person who has considerable intellectual, psychological and physical agility. Not the sort of person who you would expect to find wondering aimlessly in the woods and unable to recognise his own wife. This is exactly what happened to him after taking a statin drug called *Lipitor*.

After taking Lipitor for just six weeks, Dr Graveline experienced *transient global amnesia (TGA)*: a sudden episode of memory loss. During an episode of TGA the recall of recent events simply vanishes, so the person cannot remember where they are or how they got there. An episode of TGA may only last for a few hours but once it has subsided, the person will not remember what happened during the episode and in some cases for a few hours before it. Suffers may also forget things that happened a day, month, or year ago.

Amnesia is not listed as a side effect of statins, but Dr Graveline suspected the drug as the cause since this was a new medicine for him and he had never experienced any of these symptoms prior to taking it. For one year Dr Graveline did not take the drug and he had no re-occurrence of the amnesia. Then after his next astronaut physical his NASA doctors suggested that he started taking the drug again. After six weeks of being back on Lipitor he had his second attack of TGA.

After his experiences Dr Graveline investigated further the link between statins and memory problems. He found hundreds of case reports from distraught patients and relatives, and even doctors. They described a full array of cognitive side effects, from amnesia and severe memory loss to confusion and disorientation – all associated with the use of statins (17).

Other studies in the scientific literature provide further evidence of a link between statins and cognitive impairment (18, 19). One study found that the use of statins was associated with manifestations of severe irritability, homicidal impulses, threats to others, road rage, generation of fear in family members, and damage to property. In each case the personality disruption was sustained until the statin was discontinued. After the drug was stopped the symptoms resolved promptly (20).

Studies have found evidence that statins can also cause erectile dysfunction (21), and a reduction in libido (22). The authors concluded that this may be caused by low testosterone levels, mainly due to cholesterol depletion by statins (22).

Birth Defects

The British Heart Foundation state that pregnant women should not take statins. This is probably as a result of studies showing that babies exposed to statins in the womb are at greater risk of suffering central nervous system defects and limb deformities. Some authors have highlighted the potential problems that can occur if the embryo does not get enough cholesterol in early pregnancy for normal development (23). Unfortunately, many women do not know they are pregnant until these vital first few weeks of the pregnancy have expired (6).

Muscle Pain, Weakness and Rhabdomyolysis

All of the statin drugs are associated with disease of the muscles. The most common adverse effects reported include muscle pain or weakness however this can in rare cases lead to *rhabdomyolysis* (11, 24). Rhabdomyolysis is the breakdown of muscle fibers resulting in the release of muscle fiber contents (*myoglobin*) into the bloodstream, which are harmful to the kidney and sometimes prove fatal.

It is extremely difficult to establish the incidence of muscle rated problems amongst people who take statins, however the number of documented cases suggest that muscle pain and fatigue often go undetected in the general clinical population and merit further study (24).

These adverse effects seem to be worse if higher doses of the statin drug are used (25), and are a particular risk when the person is also taking other medications (26). This is an important consideration because it has been suggested that for some people, higher doses of statins should be used in order to reduce LDL levels considerably lower than the current target (27).

Exercise also seems to exacerbate symptoms of muscle pain and weakness (28, 29). This is of concern because a person taking statins will be less likely to exercise if it causes an increase in adverse effects, and therefore they will be much less likely to make appropriate lifestyle changes to reduce their risk for heart disease.

CHAPTER 11

New Perspectives on
Heart Disease

There are many different types of heart disease, however, the type
that kills most people is called *atherosclerosis*. Atherosclerosis is not
so much a disease of the heart: rather, it affects the arteries that
supply blood to the heart. The progression of atherosclerosis
involves the build up of various substances in the artery walls.
These substances gradually become thicker and eventually start to
harden to form hard deposits that are called *plaques*.

The thickening and hardening process involved in the formation
of a plaque is believed to take a number of years to develop. While
this is happening, *scar tissue* forms and can rupture. Scar tissue is
fibrous tissue formed as a result of wound healing - it restricts
normal elasticity of tissue. When scar tissue ruptures the body
responds by causing blood to *clot*.

These blood clots (or *thrombi*) may block the artery at the site of
injury or break away, travel through the blood vessels and get
jammed elsewhere. The tissues downstream of the blockage get
starved of oxygen.

If this is an artery supplying the heart muscle, then the result will
be a heart attack (technically known as a *myocardial infarction*).

The arteries that supply blood and oxygen to the heart are known as *coronary arteries*: hence the term *coronary heart disease (CHD)*. The same condition is sometimes referred to as *coronary artery disease (CAD)*, and falls into the general category of *cardiovascular disease (CVD)*. CVD is the name given to any dysfunction of the heart or blood vessels. For our purposes, we can think of heart disease, atherosclerosis, CHD and CAD as the same condition and all being forms of CVD.

As a result of the way that heart disease is portrayed, most people are still being misled about the fundamental mechanism of the disease. It was previously thought that saturated fat and cholesterol simply get stuck to the artery walls and 'clog them up' because there is too much of these substances in the bloodstream. However, we now know that this description does not match the reality of what happens.

In humans, the build up of plaques and the resulting narrowing of the arteries actually occurs within the wall of the artery: between the inside and outside walls of the artery. This is shown in figure 11A. It is important to state here that this is known to be fact and there are not any experts who would disagree with this. Unfortunately many organisations have *stuck* to the old model when describing heart disease to the general public, and this is keeping many misconceptions alive.

At the site of atherosclerosis and the resulting plaque formation, a whole range of different substances are found. Yes, fat and cholesterol are present, but along with a number of other substances such as *monocytes* and *macrophages*. These are white blood cells that are associated with inflammation. *Cytokines* are also found that have specific effects on cell to cell interaction. So too are *T lymphocytes*, which are white blood cells that increase in the presence of an infection (1).

The process involved in atherosclerosis was considered to be mostly due to the accumulation of fats within the artery wall: however, it is much more than that. In fact the tissue damage that is found in atherosclerosis represents a series of highly specific cellular and molecular responses that can be best described as an inflammatory disease (2). These comments were made by Dr Russell Ross from the University of Washington in an article published in the *New England Journal of Medicine*. It is worth noting that this article was published in 1999, providing an indication of the reluctance the medical community has exhibited in the acceptance of these facts.

But Doesn't Cholesterol Block Arteries?

It is said that when cholesterol levels are high, cholesterol passes from the bloodstream into the inner lining of an artery, causing atherosclerosis and eventually impeding blood flow. It is true that cholesterol is found within artery walls that have atherosclerosis: however it does not automatically follow that the cholesterol has been deposited there simply because there are higher levels of cholesterol in the blood.

If there was a simple connection in this respect, we would expect to find that people who have atherosclerosis have higher blood cholesterol levels than people who do not. From chapter 5, we already know that most people who have heart disease actually have lower cholesterol levels. Further evidence that high cholesterol does not cause atherosclerosis has been established by Uffe Ravnskov, an independent researcher from Sweden.

Dr Ravnskov has investigated all of the studies that have looked at cholesterol and atherosclerosis (3). His analysis shows that there is no correlation between more cholesterol in the bloodstream and the amount of atherosclerosis in the arteries.

Dr Ravnskov also cites the example of calcium and kidney stones: which is an example of a situation, where the level of a substance in the blood is not related to deposits of that substance in a particular location within the body.

Kidney stones are small, solid masses that form when salts (minerals) become solid crystals inside the kidney; these can build up inside the kidney and form much larger stones. Kidney stones are mostly made up of calcium: however no-one believes that high blood levels of calcium cause them to occur. A range of other potential reasons exist why these deposits occur. But it is fully accepted that they have nothing at all to do with circulating levels of calcium in the bloodstream. It is recognised that calcium is a vital substance within the body and the mechanisms involved in the development of kidney stones are more complicated than a simple build up of excess calcium.

In the same way that excess blood levels of calcium do not cause kidney stones, it is also true that higher levels of cholesterol in the blood do not cause plaques in arteries.

Heart Disease Is Inflammatory

It is now almost universally accepted that the development of atherosclerosis starts with some kind of tissue damage and inflammation plays a key role in the building up of plaques in arteries (2, 4 -12). Some researchers have stated that this new information represents a "paradigm shift in our understanding" of the events leading up to symptoms of heart disease (7) and "over

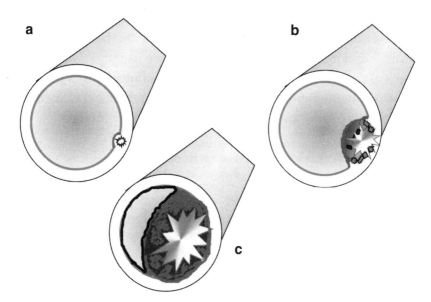

Figure 11A. Illustrating the build up of a plaque during atherosclerosis. The process starts with tissue injury that occurs underneath the inside wall of the artery (a). Then a wide range of different substances are sent to the site of injury (b). If damage to the area continues, plaque builds up and eventually starts to narrow the artery by reducing the internal diameter (c). During this process blood clots can form.

the past decade, the importance of inflammation in the development of atherosclerosis has become clear" (10). The contemporary view of atherosclerosis has "broadened to include an active and complex role for inflammation" (11). In fact, the earliest type of tissue damage (the so called *fatty streak*) is a pure inflammatory type of injury (2).

The inflammation that occurs during atherosclerosis is very much the same as the type of inflammation that we experience, for example, in the case of a sprained ankle joint, pulled muscle, or other structural injury. In the case of this type of injury we are fully aware of it and we know that if we rest the affected area it will normally repair itself after a few days. However in the case of tissue damage and inflammation in the arteries, we usually have no idea that it is taking place. Therefore we may continue doing what ever is causing or aggravating the inflammation, until one day we start to experience symptoms or in the worse case, a heart attack.

Inflammation is a local reaction to injury. Although it can occur almost anywhere in the body and can take many forms, the type of reaction is always the same. When a child develops a sore throat, microbes have proliferated in the tonsils causing local swelling. This inflammation of the tonsils is of course called *tonsillitis*. If microbes get out of control in the appendix and cause swelling we call it *appendicitis*. Inflammation of the liver is called *hepatitis*, of the kidney *nephritis* and of the joints is *arthritis* (13). Perhaps in the future, heart disease will be known as *coronary arteritis*, although this may not describe the complete process, it does depict the condition in a more meaningful and accurate way than the simple 'artery clogging' description.

The term *coronary arteritis* may encourage the investigation into alternative treatment protocols for heart disease and help to put the role of saturated fat and cholesterol into context.

In fact, heart disease has been compared with rheumatoid arthritis, a condition that also has key inflammatory and immune system components. Some researchers have studied the similarities between atherosclerosis and rheumatoid arthritis in an attempt to better understand how heart disease develops. A remarkable pattern of similarity emerges between the two diseases, in that both have evidence for activation of various cells associated with the immune system and inflammation. Both diseases also involve activation of *endothelial cells* (14).

Our arteries actually 'feel' the blood flowing through them. The sensors that read how hard the blood pushes and pulls as it rushes through the body are called endothelial cells. These cells line the inside wall of the arteries and are alive in their own right (15). Endothelial cells were previously thought to consist of a passive membrane or layer: however more recent knowledge has shown that they perform a number of very important and complex tasks. They also have the ability to adapt to specific needs in time and location. Inflammation, artery wall re-modelling, the release of immune factors and the regulation of the tone of the arteries are some of the functions undertaken by endothelial cells. They are generally associated with keeping everything balanced and under control in the blood vessels and arteries.

Endothelial cells coordinate the recruitment of inflammatory cells to sites of tissue injury or infection (16). Of course, something has to happen to cause this initial injury or infection, and it is extremely unlikely to be simply caused by the presence of cholesterol in the blood (which should be there anyway!). There are many things that can cause the initial tissue damage leading to inflammation and there are many factors that may contribute to the continued development of atherosclerosis. These causes and contributing factors include:

High Levels of Stress / Poor Stress Response
Wrong Balance or 'Mix' of Foods
Eating too Many 'Grain-based Foods
High Blood Glucose Levels
Eating too Many Refined Foods and Sugars
High Blood Pressure
Low-Thyroid Function / Adrenal Gland Exhaustion
Hormonal Imbalances
Exercise: Wrong Type or Amount for Individual Person

Processed and De-natured Foods
Psychology: Depression, Attitude
Lack of Protective Nutrients
Excessive Toxins
Infection
Lack of Sleep

In previous chapters we have seen that cholesterol is the substance that provides integrity to cells: making them waterproof, protecting them from the local external environment. Is it not possible that the cholesterol found at the site of tissue damage and inflammation is present in an attempt to re-build the damaged cells?

The treatment of high cholesterol levels and high blood pressure was expected to eliminate heart disease by the end of the 20th century. However, the continued high incidence of the disease has forced us to consider new strategies for prediction, prevention and treatment (4).

Better Ways to Measure Heart Disease Risk

There are in fact a number of other parameters or markers that can be used to estimate the risk of heart disease and some of these are more accurate, not to mention more appropriate, than cholesterol levels. Emerging risk factors or markers that researchers have identified include (adapted from reference 17):

- Estrogen deficiency
- Homocysteine
- Plasma fibrinogen
- Factor VII
- Endogenous tissue plasminogen activator

- Plasminogen-activator inhibitor type 1
- D-Dimer
- Lipoprotein(a)
- C-reactive protein
- Chlamydia pneumoniae

The intention here is not to provide a detailed discussion of each of these but to highlight two of the markers which are highly significant for our discussion. These are *C-Reactive Protein* and *Homocysteine*.

C-Reactive Protein, Inflammation and Statins

As we shall see in chapter 13, when cholesterol lowering drugs (statins) do show any benefit, the effects are usually exaggerated. In addition to this, any benefits are most likely to be due to other effects that have nothing to do with cholesterol.

C-Reactive Protein (CRP) is an amino acid that is produced by the liver. It is a measurable substance that directly relates to the amount of inflammation within the body. When there is acute inflammation within the body the amount of CRP tends to increase. CRP is emerging as the best marker for inflammation and a very important risk factor for heart disease (4-8, 10, 18 -21). Numerous studies have shown that cholesterol lowering drugs (statins) reduce inflammation and in many of these studies the reduction in inflammation is independent of any effects on cholesterol levels (22). This means that any benefit provided by statins could be related to the reduction in inflammation rather than the effects on cholesterol.

The reader will recall from chapter 8 that Statins block all biochemical reactions downstream from a specific point in the production of cholesterol. This means that a large number of other substances cannot be produced within the body. Imagine a toy factory that makes a range of different toys but all from the same type of plastic – if the plastic is not available none of the toys can be manufactured. Inflammatory molecules are one of the substances that depend on the same raw material as cholesterol. Statins prevent the production of this raw material and block the progression of inflammation.

A study published in the journal *Circulation*, investigated the use of a cholesterol lowering drug in people who had already had a heart attack. The authors also investigated the possibility that inflammation increases the risk of having future coronary events. A coronary event generally speaking is a term used to describe a wide range of heart problems and includes heart attacks.

This study found that there was a 28% reduced risk of a future coronary event in the people who were given the statin. However, there were large differences in the benefits achieved depending on the presence of inflammation. Among those with evidence of inflammation, the use of the statin prevented 54% of future coronary events compared with just 25% among those without inflammation. This was despite the fact that levels of total cholesterol, LDL 'cholesterol', and HDL 'cholesterol', were the same in those with and those without evidence of inflammation (23). This shows that any benefits that the statin drug provided were associated with the reduction in inflammation and other effects that are not related to cholesterol lowering.

A study published in the *New England Journal of Medicine* investigated the use of a statin drug in 3,745 patients with an existing heart condition. The authors concluded that patients who had low C-Reactive Protein levels after using the statin had better clinical outcomes than those with higher C-Reactive Protein levels. This was regardless of the resulting level of LDL 'cholesterol' (20).

Researchers from the Cleveland Clinic in America have published a review article (24) of the Heart Protection Study (25). This study included 20,536 men and women aged 40 to 80 years who were considered to have an increased risk of death from heart disease within 5 years. The authors suggest that the Heart Protection Study makes a strong argument for the widespread use of statin drugs. They suggest that statins are underused and increasing their use would significantly reduce the worldwide burden of cardiovascular disease.

By looking at the results of the Heart Protection Study we can clearly see that 12.9% of the people treated with the statin died, verses 14.7% of people who were not treated with the statin – a risk reduction of just 1.8%. As we have already seen in chapter 10, statins have a number of potentially very serious side effects. It is questionable that people would want to expose themselves to the risks associated with these side effects and the burden of taking daily medication for the rest of their lives along with regular tests and visits to their doctor, for a mere 1.8% reduction in the risk of dieing from cardiovascular disease.

What is even more intriguing with the Heart Protection Study, (as stated by Dr Uffe Ravnskov in a letter to the *British Medical Journal*) is that the effect of the statin was independent of the cholesterol level. The patients with low cholesterol benefited just as much (or as little) as patients with high cholesterol (26).

This again provides more evidence that any benefits that statins do provide have nothing to do with cholesterol lowering. Dr

Ravnskov has also pointed out that the greatest benefits from the statin drug were experienced by patients older than 75 years. As discussed in chapter 7, the evidence clearly shows that reducing cholesterol in this age group actually increases the risk of death. The fact that statins provided more benefit for this age group than other age groups yet again tells us that any benefits cannot be associated with cholesterol levels.

Another study published in the *New England Journal of Medicine* measured the C-Reactive Protein and LDL 'cholesterol' levels in 27,939 healthy women. The women were followed for eight years in order to compare the ability of these two substances to predict cardiovascular problems such as a heart attack or stroke. The researchers found that C-Reactive Protein was a stronger predictor, and better for assessing risk than LDL 'cholesterol' (18).

One study found that statins reduce the level of C-Reactive Protein within just 14 days and this again was independent of the reduction in the level of LDL 'cholesterol' (27). Another study found that a statin drug provided significant improvement in people with the inflammatory disease: rheumatoid arthritis (28).

Some people may be of the opinion that it does not really matter that much if any benefit is associated with inflammation, other effects, or cholesterol. However, as discussed in chapter 8, statins are extremely expensive and cost billions of pounds. When we recognise that the benefits are largely associated with other effects than cholesterol we can, in many cases, investigate alternative treatment protocols, which may save the tax payer hundreds of millions of pounds. In addition, we must accurately identify where benefits are being derived so that we can improve future therapeutic methods. Not to mention the fact that we will then be able to finally put an end to the billions of pounds that is being wasted on trying to 'prove' the cholesterol idea. This money could be used for research into finding effective medications for a real disease rather than a fictitious risk factor.

Dr McCully Is Finally Vindicated

Dr Kilmer McCully was a highly respected physician at Harvard University and the Massachusetts General Hospital. In 1968 he discovered a link between a substance called *homocysteine* and heart disease. Homocysteine is a protein that is normally found in the blood in small quantities. Dr McCully discovered that when the amount of homocysteine in the blood gets too high, it can damage the arteries and cause or contribute to heart disease. The most interesting and useful part of his discovery is that homocysteine tends to be too high when there is a deficiency of the nutrients *folic acid*, *vitamin B12* and *vitamin B6*. Generally speaking, the level of homocysteine can be reduced by increasing the intake of these nutrients.

When Dr McCully began publishing his work on homocysteine in the 1970s, the cholesterol idea was already taking momentum and several government agencies in America were already gearing-up for a national education program to make cholesterol a national preoccupation. Few people wanted to hear about the discovery of the homocysteine–heart disease link, since this clearly put the cholesterol idea onto the 'backburners' and so many people had already committed a lot of time and money into trying to 'prove' cholesterol is the villain. Perhaps more significantly: homocysteine could be lowered through diet or inexpensive nutritional supplements, but cholesterol had to be lowered through the use of very expensive drugs. Thus making the homocysteine theory much less attractive to powerful pharmaceutical companies.

In 1970, Dr McCully was praised by a special Scientific Advisory Committee at Massachusetts General Hospital for his work and important contributions on homocysteine. However as time went by the people at the top of the hospital became less interested in the homocysteine theory and eventually McCully was forced to leave his position.

For two years after, McCully was unable to get a job anywhere and he began to hear about phone calls from Harvard that were discrediting his character. This prompted him to take legal action. Only after taking these steps did he find a new position at a different institution.

Dr McCully has now finally been vindicated and homocysteine has now been widely accepted as an emerging risk factor for heart disease. These discoveries are summarised in his book *The Heart Revolution* (29).

The extent of the role that homocysteine plays in the overall complex puzzle of heart disease still has to be fully explored. The routine screening of homocysteine levels and the amount of risk homocysteine levels represent still has to be further investigated (30). An analysis published in the *British Medical Journal* looked at a number of studies that have been completed on homocysteine and concluded that there was strong evidence for the link between homocysteine and heart disease (31).

Researchers at Tufts University, Boston studied 1160 adults between the ages of 67 and 96 years. They found that 29.3% of people in this age group had high homocysteine levels, and high homocysteine was found most often in people with low levels of folic acid. In addition, low levels of one or more B vitamins appeared to contribute to 67% of the cases of high homocysteine (32).

Incidentally, animal proteins containing saturated fats (exactly the foods we are told to avoid) are the best dietary sources of the B vitamins that can help to keep homocysteine at the appropriate level.

Oxidised Cholesterol

This chapter would not be complete without briefly mentioning *oxidised cholesterol*, which is very different from normal cholesterol. Unfortunately researchers do not always differentiate between normal cholesterol and oxidised cholesterol and this often leads to misunderstandings.

Cholesterol can react with oxygen to become *oxidised* in the body. *Antioxidants* are believed to protect cholesterol from becoming oxidised. As discussed in chapter 10, antioxidants are natural substances that exist as vitamins, minerals and other compounds. They act as *electron donors* and deactivate *free radicals*, preventing free radicals from injuring cells.

LDLs carry their own antioxidants but if there are fewer antioxidants available, the cholesterol attached to the LDL particle may become oxidised. Oxidised cholesterol can injure endothelial cells and trigger or contribute to the process of atherosclerosis (4, 7). It is therefore very important to minimise the number of oxidised LDLs within the body.

The consumption of too much polyunsaturated fat (referred to as 'good' fats by dieticians and the food industry) leads to greater numbers of free radicals within the body and potentially greater numbers of oxidised LDLs, On the other hand, saturated fats help prevent LDLs from becoming oxidised because these fats are more stable and less likely to generate free radicals. Also, as discussed in chapter 10, statins may reduce the availability of some vitally important antioxidants needed to protect cholesterol from oxidation.

CHAPTER 12

More on Glucose, Diabetes and Heart Disease

In chapter 3 we discussed some of the problems associated with the consumption of too much carbohydrate and more specifically the dangers associated with increasing the intake of grain based foods, such as bread, rice, breakfast cereals and pasta. It was shown that these foods cause the levels of glucose (sugar) in the blood to significantly increase and numerous studies have demonstrated that high blood glucose increases the risk for disease. Armed with this knowledge and information gained from the intermediary chapters of this book we are now able to discuss in more detail how excess carbohydrate consumption and the resulting high blood glucose levels are related to diabetes and heart disease.

Before, going into more detail about the adverse effects caused by high blood glucose, let us briefly look at the problems with the conventional view of diabetes. Diabetes in this chapter, refers to *type 2 diabetes* (as described in chapter 3), which accounts for around 90% of all the people diagnosed with diabetes.

What's Wrong with the Conventional View of Diabetes?

Diabetes is reaching epidemic proportions and affects more than 170 million people worldwide. Global estimates for the year 2010 predict that this number will increase by almost 50% (1) and that

300 million people will have diabetes by the year 2025 (2). Despite the fact that diabetes is rapidly increasing in many countries, there appears to be very little effort directed towards finding out what causes the disease. As with heart disease, most of the resources available for research into diabetes have been focussed on risk factors for the disease and the testing of new drugs for the condition: rather than being directed toward the cause itself. The information we are given about the actual cause of diabetes is vague and the dietary advice given to diabetics is full of contradictions.

The conventional view of diabetes is that it is caused by a "combination of genetic and environmental factors" (3). Namely: age, family history, ethnic origin, being overweight, and having a waist circumference greater than a specified size (4). Experts seldom discuss the actual causes but focus instead on the above risk factors. Of course, the only two of these risk factors that can be modified are body weight and waist circumference. Therefore from a lifestyle management point of view, attention is directed towards weight management through diet and physical activity (5).

Obesity and diabetes are so often seen together that some experts have coined the term "diabesity" (6). However it is worth mentioning that this is a mathematical link. Being overweight or obese may contribute to diabetes but it is not described as the main cause. As stated above, there is little attention given to trying to find the cause.

In some ways, it is convenient to focus on the likelihood that someone who is overweight will also be diabetic. This makes it easier to find customers for diabetes drugs – all that has to be done is to advertise for people who have a waist circumference above a certain size. In effect, this is the best demographic of the target market for diabetes drugs.

An extensive campaign organised by Diabetes UK (www.diabetes.org.uk) has been running throughout 2007 and 2008 in the UK called the "Measure Up" campaign. This campaign urges people with two or more risk factors for diabetes to get a test for diabetes. The main risk factor that is emphasised in this campaign is waist circumference. Figure 12A shows one of the images that have been used as part of the Measure Up campaign. This image formed the basis of adverts that were placed on the side of bus shelters across London. It was also used for double page adverts in newspapers.

The real value of the Measure Up campaign has to be questioned. Once people have responded to these advertisements and had a test for diabetes, those who are diagnosed with the condition are likely to be prescribed diabetes medications. In addition, they may be advised to follow a low fat/ high carbohydrate diet. It is clear that this type of diet can have adverse effects for people with diabetes. A cynic may suggest that there is little incentive to recognise this fact since the recommended low fat/high carbohydrate diet is likely to ensure the continued growth of the market for diabetes drugs.

It could be argued that the Measure Up campaign has raised public awareness of diabetes. Diabetes UK has claimed that the campaign has reduced the incidence of complications associated with diabetes. This may be true but surely Diabetes UK should also be looking into what is causing the diabetes epidemic rather than accepting it and merely finding those who are eligible for diabetes drugs.

Where is the campaign for the prevention of diabetes? If a person has already gained a considerable amount of weight and has other risk factors, they may already be well on their way to a diagnosis

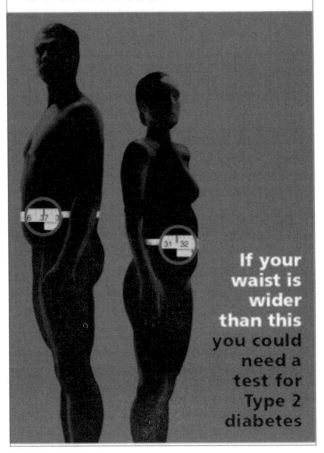

Figure 12A. An Image Used as Part of the
Diabetes UK "Measure Up" Campaign.

of diabetes. Why are people not told about the dangers associated with high blood glucose levels? Why are people not told about the studies referenced in chapter 3 showing that high blood glucose (even below the diabetic threshold) is associated with a greater number of deaths from any cause? Why are people not informed that high blood glucose represents around the same level of risk for heart disease as does smoking cigarettes? Why are more people not being screened for high blood glucose before the level reaches that associated with diabetes? These are the areas that need to be addressed if we really want to counteract the diabetes epidemic. But we are not informing people about these facts – perhaps because some organisations are more interested in the business opportunities provided by the expanding diabetes market?

As indicated above, the diet that is recommended to diabetics is low in fat and high in carbohydrate (7). It is believed that a low fat diet will help diabetics to lose weight. However, there are no studies to demonstrate that this type of diet is beneficial for diabetics. This advice is based on the assumption that dietary fat causes weight gain. But, as we have already seen in chapter 3, there are numerous studies to show that a low fat / high carbohydrate diet is more likely to lead to weight gain. The potential problems associated with this kind of diet are particularly relevant to diabetics. Since diabetics by definition have high blood glucose levels – resulting in high levels of the hormone *insulin*, which blocks the ability to 'burn' stored body fat.

The low fat / high carbohydrate diet, for many people, is a major contributing factor to the development of diabetes. It is exactly the type of diet that for a large number of people, will lead to the continued progression of the condition. It also increases the risk for further complications.

It is absurd that diabetics are advised to eat starchy foods like bread, rice and pasta. As we have seen in chapter 3, these are the worst foods we can eat if we are trying to get control over blood glucose levels!

In terms of medication, one of the main aims for the treatment of diabetes is to manage blood glucose levels (5). A range of blood glucose lowering drugs are used, but unfortunately some of these actually cause further weight gain (1, 2).

Another aim of drug treatment is to lower total cholesterol levels and 'bad' cholesterol (LDLs). It is assumed that lowering cholesterol will reduce the increased risk that diabetics have for developing heart disease. However, people with diabetes do not have increased LDL 'cholesterol' levels (8). It is common to find normal or average LDL levels in people who are diabetic (9) and in fact, total cholesterol tends to be low (10).

A vast array of self help books have been published on diabetes. Some of these books suggest that cholesterol levels are high in people who have diabetes. If we compare the cholesterol levels found in people who have diabetes with the targets that have been set (5mmol/l or total cholesterol and 3mmol/l for LDLs), then we may conclude that cholesterol is high in people who have diabetes. However, the fact is that most of the non-diabetic population in the UK have cholesterol levels above these arbitrary values. It is important to compare cholesterol levels with the rest of the population in order to determine if they are high in people with diabetes. When we do this we consistently find that cholesterol is not high in people with diabetes, and in fact very often it is lower than the average level.

The abnormalities in diabetes are not associated with total

cholesterol or the level of LDLs. There are other abnormalities that are much more relevant and pose a much greater risk. These are discussed below.

High Carbohydrate Diet Increases Triglycerides

When we eat too much carbohydrate, blood glucose levels increase rapidly. Since high blood glucose levels are very dangerous and can cause considerable damage within the body, this excess glucose has to be converted into fat. The type of fat that is made from glucose is called a *triglyceride*. Therefore a diet that contains too much carbohydrate leads to high levels of triglycerides in the blood. Numerous studies have found that a low fat / high carbohydrate diet causes high blood levels of triglycerides (11-21) and a high level of triglycerides is an extremely common characteristic of diabetes (22, 23).

High levels of triglycerides in the blood cause levels of HDLs (so called 'good' cholesterol) to be lowered. This is why high levels of triglycerides and low levels of HDLs are so often found together (24). Along with high triglycerides, diabetics almost always have low levels of HDLs (22, 23). It is also a well established fact that a high carbohydrate diet causes low levels of HDLs (11, 12, 14, 16, 18, 19, 21, 25-27).

LDL Particle Size

Another abnormality that is found in people who have diabetes is related to the actual size of LDL particles. This issue is not related to the level or number of LDLs within the blood, but is associated with the diameter of the LDLs that do exist. People with diabetes have smaller LDLs (22, 23). As LDLs become smaller in size their properties change considerably and their effects can be very different from larger or normal size LDLs.

Readers will recall from the previous chapter that when heart disease is present, fat and cholesterol do not simply get stuck to the inside wall of an artery. Rather, tissue damage occurs beneath the inside wall of an artery and a process of inflammation commences. When LDLs are smaller in diameter, they can pass through the inside wall of an artery much more easily. They can also more easily become oxidised and cause further tissue damage. In fact, there are at least eight different mechanisms where by LDLs can become dangerous when they are reduced in size (24).

It is now widely recognised that smaller LDL particles are associated with a greater risk for heart disease (28-30), and larger LDLs are associated with a longer life (31). A diet that is higher in saturated fat actually increases the size of LDL particles (32, 33) and a high carbohydrate/low saturated fat diet leads to a smaller LDL particle size (25, 34-36). These facts alone are sufficient to prove that a low fat/ high carbohydrate diet is detrimental for people who have diabetes, and also for the general population. However, the evidence against a low fat/ high carbohydrate diet does not stop there.

The resulting high blood glucose levels from the consumption of too much carbohydrate actually damages our arteries.

Cholesterol Levels Found in Diabetes - Summary

Diabetics have normal, or slightly low total cholesterol levels, and normal or average levels of LDLs. The metabolic abnormalities that are of concern in people with diabetes are:

- a high level of triglycerides
- low levels of HDLs
- a small LDL particle size

Studies have repeatedly shown that a low fat / high carbohydrate diet causes all of these abnormalities.

Having a low level of HDLs is not necessarily a problem in itself, but it is an effect of having high triglycerides. The high level of triglycerides and the small LDL particle size are two of the important factors that increase the risk for heart disease.

How High Glucose Damages Arteries

Our blood vessels and arteries are dynamic. They are in a constant state of change and adapt to the demands that are put upon them. The changes that occur are controlled by *endothelial cells*. These cells line the inside wall of the blood vessels and arteries and perform a wide range of different tasks. They generally keep everything within vessels and arteries balanced and under control. The presence of too much glucose in the blood can actually impair the normal functioning of the endothelial cells (37-41). In particular, high blood glucose can prevent blood vessels from dilating (widening). This has very important implications for the flow of blood and oxygen through the blood vessels to the heart.

Endothelial cells synthesise a substance called *nitric oxide*. This substance actually causes blood vessels to widen so that blood can flow through more easily (38). High levels of blood glucose can actually inhibit the ability of endothelial cells to manufacture nitric oxide (38, 40, 41). Further more: nitric oxide is also involved in a number of other functions that protect against heart disease (38).

Overall, problems with the functioning of endothelial cells form a key step in the progression of heart disease (41). It is well established that people with diabetes have an impaired endothelial cell function (42), but studies have also shown that these problems can occur in people who have just slightly high blood glucose levels, considerably lower than the levels associated with diabetes (41).

These are just some of the explanations why high blood glucose levels have repeatedly been shown to increase the risk for heart disease. As discussed in chapter 3, there is a gradual relationship between blood glucose levels and heart disease, even below the threshold for diabetes. Further evidence for this was established by researchers who looked at 20 published studies on this subject, involving 95,783 people. The authors concluded: "the progressive relationship between glucose levels and cardiovascular risk extends below the diabetic threshold" (43).

Some studies have shown that the addition of certain nutrients such as vitamin E can actually protect endothelial cells from the damage caused by high blood glucose levels (41). Readers will recall from chapter 11 that vitamin E is carried through the blood by LDLs and HDLs. Remember also that cholesterol is vital for the repair of cells which may have been damaged by high levels of blood glucose. Therefore, it is feasible that total cholesterol levels, along with LDL and HDL levels are altered in the presence of high blood glucose – but as part of the protective mechanisms of the body.

An interesting point arises related to gender differences in diabetes and heart disease. Women who have diabetes are more likely than men with diabetes to develop heart disease (44). Some studies have shown that women may be more susceptible to the lowering of HDLs that is caused by high blood glucose levels (since a low fat / high carbohydrate diet seems to lower HDLs more in women than in men) (26). We also know that in men, more vitamin E is carried in LDLs, but in women, more vitamin E is carried in HDLs (45). Therefore, the availability of vitamin E may be reduced more in women than in men when blood glucose levels are high. Vitamin E not only protects endothelial cells but can also prevent damage to other substances within the body. This potential greater reduction in the availability of vitamin E in women may be one explanation why diabetes can lead to heart disease more frequently in women.

High Glucose and Inflammation

Inflammation is a major part of the development of heart disease. In the previous chapter, the term *coronary arteritis* was coined to emphasise the importance of inflammation in heart disease. Studies have clearly shown that a diet that is high in carbohydrate content increases inflammation (46). Other studies have shown that inflammation is reduced by increasing the protein and fat content of the diet (47).

In order to determine the level of inflammation within the body, researchers' measure a substance called *C-Reactive Protein (CRP)*. High levels of CRP are associated with a significantly increased risk for heart disease. CRP drastically increases when the *glycemic load* of the diet increases (46). The glycemic load is related to the carbohydrate content of the diet. It signifies the extent that the diet will raise blood glucose levels. Generally, the higher the carbohydrate content of the diet, the higher the glycemic load will be. This increase in CRP associated with increasing glycemic load could theoretically translate to a 60% increased risk for heart disease (46).

The Status Quo May Just be Too Convenient

This chapter, along with chapter 3 raises important questions about the information the authorities provide us with about diabetes. The available evidence is contrary to the dietary advice that is given to people who have diabetes and those who wish to prevent it. In fact, current guidelines are more likely to increase the risk for diabetes. When we look at the research, the inappropriateness of a low fat/high carbohydrate diet for people with diabetes becomes obvious. So obvious that it raises questions about the motivations behind these recommendations. There is no evidence of direct deception, but it has to be said that there is a lot to be gained by continuing with the status quo.

Drugs for treating diabetes represent one of the fastest growing markets for the pharmaceutical industry and several companies are developing new drugs for this market.

Drugs such as *SGLT2 Inhibitors* and *DPP-4 Inhibitors* are designed to help control blood glucose levels in one way or another (48, 49). Several new drugs are being developed that fall into this category, but few people are told that blood glucose can often be controlled by simple dietary changes. Some of the new drugs are predicted to generate US$2 billion in sales per year each (50). The financial press has commented that the diabetes market is big enough to have more than one blockbuster drug (50).

CHAPTER 13

Cholesterol Drugs on Trial

Considering the enthusiasm that much of the medical community has for cholesterol lowering drugs (statins), we may assume that a huge body of evidence exists to prove that these drugs provide significant benefits for the people who take them. Statins have been portrayed as a kind of wonder drug or "the pill of life" (1). Unfortunately, the claims that are made about these drugs are routinely exaggerated and summary information from clinical trials is all too often carefully written to imply much more overall benefit than was actually achieved. This chapter briefly discusses some of the clinical trials and larger studies that have been completed on statins. The intention is to provide readers with a realistic impression of the effectiveness of statins. Then, armed with the information contained in chapter 10 about potential side effects, an informed choice can be made about the risk / benefit balance associated with the life-time use of these drugs.

The AFCAPS/TexCAPS Trial

The AFCAPS/TexCAPS trial included 5608 men and 997 women with average cholesterol levels and no existing signs of cardiovascular disease (2). The aim of the trial was to test if a cholesterol lowering statin was able to reduce the number of first coronary events (for example, a first heart attack) in this group of people. Researchers call this *primary prevention*. This trial is of interest because the group of people included are similar to many of those who are prescribed statins under the guidelines doctors are working to in 2008.

After just over five years, the group of people who were given the statin had fewer heart attacks. However, in terms of percentages: 3.3% of the statin group had a heart attack verses 5.6% of the placebo group: a difference of just 2.3%.

What is of more concern, however, is whether or not the statin drug actually saved any lives. In the summary of the trial report the authors' state: "there were no clinically relevant differences in safety parameters between treatment groups". Unfortunately they fail to mention here the fact that overall, slightly more people died in the group given the statin (80 people) than those not given the drug (77 people).

Although the use of the statin significantly reduced LDL 'cholesterol', and was associated with less cardiovascular related deaths, more people died from other causes. In the statin group 63 people died from other causes, verses 52 in the placebo group. This did not however, stop the authors from stating that this study confirmed the benefits of reducing LDL 'cholesterol'. It should be no surprise that this study was funded by one of the statin manufacturers (Merck & Co Inc.), who also employed some of the authors.

The ASCOT-LLA Trial

This was another primary prevention trial to test the effects of lowering cholesterol with a statin. It included 10,305 people (mostly men) aged 40 to 79 years, with high blood pressure or other risk factors for cardiovascular disease, but with average cholesterol levels (3). As with the study described above, the people included in this trial are typical of those who could be prescribed a statin under current guidelines. The average total cholesterol level of the people included in the study was 5.5 mmol/l and the average level of LDL 'cholesterol' was 3.4 mmol/l. In 2008, the target is to have a total cholesterol level less than 5.0 mmol/l and a level of LDL 'cholesterol' below 3.0 mmol/l.

Researchers often use the term *primary end point* to describe the specific outcomes that will be measured in a trial. In this case the primary end points were a heart attack or death due to heart disease. Within the group of people who were given the statin, 1.9% of them had a heart attack or died of heart disease, verses 3% of people in the placebo group. The statin reduced the risk by just 1.1%. Unfortunately the authors of the report did not emphasise this point. Instead they described the results as a 36% reduction in primary end points. The authors calculated that the 1.1% reduction in risk between the statin and placebo groups was 36% of 3%. In other words, they used a relative percentage instead of an absolute percentage difference. This is a clever manipulation of the data. If a person is told that a statin will reduce their risk by 36%, they may be inclined to take the drug, but if they are told that in real terms, this 36% means a reduction from 3% risk to 1.9%, they may think twice about it.

It is interesting that the trial was planned to run for 5 years but the researchers were so happy with these results that they decided to stop the trial after 3.3 years. They believed that they had done enough to prove the benefits of the statin being tested.

Again, when we look at the results for deaths from all causes, 3.6% of people died in the statin group verses 4.1% in the placebo group. A reduction in the overall death rate of just 0.5% - even though LDL 'cholesterol' was significantly reduced in the statin group.

The CTT Trials

Researchers completed an overall analysis of 14 statin trials. This included 90,056 participants from a wide range of different groups. Some people in the trial had existing heart disease, other forms of cardiovascular disease, or diabetes, and others had none of these conditions (4). The aim of the trial was to investigate the effect that reducing LDL 'cholesterol' by 1 mmol/l will have on various outcomes. It should be noted that 1 mmol/l represents a large reduction in LDLs, since values are typically low anyway.

The results showed that reducing the level of LDLs by 1 mmol/l reduced the risk of dieing from heart disease from 4.4% to 3.4%. Although this study included a larger proportion of people who were at high risk for heart disease, the statin still only achieved a reduction in the risk of just 1%.

Again, when we look at death from all causes, the results are disappointing - with a death rate of 8.5% in the statin group, compared with 9.7% in the placebo group.

The same group of researchers published another study in the *Lancet* in 2008. They used the data from the trial described above, but this time more specifically looked at the people within the study who had diabetes (5). Their analysis showed that the people with diabetes benefited even less than those without diabetes. Since the statin only managed to reduce the number of deaths from all causes in diabetic people from 11.9% in the statin group to 11.0% in the placebo group. This did not stop the authors from recommending that statins should be considered for all people with diabetes.

Again, most of the trials included in this analysis were supported by grants from the pharmaceutical industry and some of the authors had their costs reimbursed by drug companies for participation at scientific meetings.

The MRC/BHF Heart Protection Study

This study included 20,536 high risk people who already had heart disease, cardiovascular disease or diabetes (6). Even in this high risk group, the use of the statin only reduced the heart disease death rate from 6.9% to 5.7% (a difference of 1.2%). The authors described this slight reduction as "highly significant".

In this study, the statin reduced the rate of death from all causes by 1.8%: from 14.7% in the placebo group to 12.9% in the statin group.

The 4S Study

The Scandinavian Simvastatin Survival Study, otherwise known as the *4S study*, was completed in 1994 and out of all the trials completed to date, has produced the best results for a statin. Numerous trials have been completed since 1994, costing billions of dollars, but none have produced the same level of results.

The 4S trial included 4,444 patients who already had heart disease, many of whom had already had a heart attack. At the end of the trial, 8% of patients in the group who were given the statin had died verses 12% of patients in the placebo group. Over 6 years, the patients in the statin group had a 91.3% probability of surviving, compared with an 87.6% probability of surviving in the placebo group (7).

The 4S trial is often quoted in support of the use of statins, but it is not always mentioned that no other trial has been able to produce the same results. Also, it is often forgotten that this trial included only very high risk patients; the results in this group can not be assumed to be the same for the general population in the prevention of a first heart attack (primary prevention). In fact, as we have seen, the benefits of statins in primary prevention have consistently been much lower.

The TNT Study

Researchers wanted to determine if increasing the dose of a statin drug would provide more benefits (8). They completed an analysis of 5,584 patients who already had heart disease and the metabolic syndrome (a condition that is similar to diabetes). 60% of the people included in this study had already had one heart attack, and more than 80% had angina (chest pain due to an inadequate supply of oxygen to the heart muscle).

One group of patients were given 10mg of a statin, and the other was given 80mg. After around 5 years, major cardiovascular problems occurred in 13% of people in the 10mg group and 9.5% of people in the 80mg group. A difference of 3.5%. Again, the authors chose to describe this as a 26% relative risk reduction (3.5% is around 26% of 13%), which is misleading to patients and doctors since it exaggerates the benefits.

In the summary report, the authors were very keen to state that increasing the dose of the statin derives "incremental benefit". They also claimed that the study provides evidence for more intensive lowering of LDL 'cholesterol' with statins for people with heart disease and metabolic syndrome. However, they failed to mention that even in this very high risk group, increasing the dose of the statin to 80mg did not make much difference to the total number of deaths. Since, 6.3% of the people in the 10mg group died of all causes, compared with 6.2% in the 80mg group.

Although LDL 'cholesterol' was lowered much more by increasing the dose of the statin, there were more deaths from non-cardiovascular causes. The slight reduction in risk of dieing from cardiovascular causes was almost outweighed by the increase in the risk of death from other causes. This study shows that lowering LDLs more intensively will not significantly increase life expectancy, even for people who are already at very high risk.

The WOSCOPS Study

The WOSCOPS study included 6,595 men in the West of Scotland, who had high cholesterol levels (9). The average total cholesterol level for the people included in the study was 7.0 mmol/l (the target, according to the supporters of the cholesterol idea is below 5.0 mmol/l). The WOSCOPS study is often used to justify the use of statins to reduce cholesterol in the general population. For example it is quoted by the British Heart Foundation as one of the "watershed studies showing significant benefits" (10). The supporters of the cholesterol idea have created an impression that having higher than average cholesterol drastically increases the risk of dieing from heart disease. However, during this five year study, 1.7% of people who were given the placebo died of heart disease, compared with 1.2% of those who were given the statin. It is also worth noting that overall, the use of the statin only increased the chances of still being alive after 5 years, from a 96% chance to a 97% chance (11).

An interesting feature of the WOSCOPS study is that around 80% of the people included were current smokers or ex-smokers. It is well known that smoking drastically increases the risk for heart disease. In fact, the heart disease death rate is 80% higher in heavy smokers than in non-smokers (12). We also know that smoking causes inflammation and this inflammation can take 5 years to return to normal levels after smoking has been stopped (13). Readers will recall from chapter 11 that heart disease is mostly an inflammatory condition and statins reduce inflammation. Therefore, any benefits that were achieved in this trial are more likely to be due to the effect the statin had on inflammation, and it is possible that this had nothing to do with cholesterol at all.

Further evidence for any benefits found in the WOSCOPS study having nothing to do with cholesterol lowering can be seen in the fact that the people in the higher band of total cholesterol level benefited less than those in the lower band. This was also the case for LDL 'cholesterol'.

The WOSCOPS Follow Up

After the initial WOSCOPS trial had been completed, researchers undertook a 10 year follow up of the trial participants (14). This follow up study was published in the *New England Journal of Medicine* – one of the most prestigious medical journals in the world. However, there are a number of serious problems with it. After the original WOSCOPS trial had been completed some of the people who were in the placebo group started taking a statin, and some of those who were in the statin group stopped taking the drug. The researchers did not take account of this in the WOSCOPS follow up study. Surely this must mean that any results obtained 10 years on are meaningless? The original groups were now mixed with some taking a statin and others not taking one.

To make matters worse, the researchers did not know how many people were taking statins after 5 years – the follow up period was 10 years but they only had data on this aspect for the first 5 years.

Even if these important issues are put to one side, the results of the study were still poor. After the 5 year period of the original WOSCOPS trial plus the 10 year follow up period (making a total of 15 years), 5.1% of the people who were originally given the statin had died of heart disease, compared with 6.3% in the original placebo group.

Another point is related to the fact that more people got cancer in the group who were originally given the statin. The authors of the study dismissed this as a chance finding. Favourable results for the statin were over-emphasised, and negative results were dismissed as unimportant. The effects that the statin had on the incidence of cancer in this study may be important because the 15 year study period is unusual for a statin trial (which is typically about 5 or 6 years in duration). Cancer does not usually appear after just 5 years, but can take decades to develop. The data from the WOSCOPS follow up period actually shows that with increasing time, people who were in the original statin group had a higher incidence of cancer than those who were not given the drug.

An accompanying editorial to this study was also published in the

New England Journal of Medicine (15).The author stated that "there should no longer be any doubt that the reduction of LDL cholesterol levels has a role in the prevention and treatment of coronary heart disease". *The Times* newspaper also featured this study in an article that took up almost a full page and was headlined on the front page. This newspaper article suggested that "statins have benefits after dosage is stopped" and that statins should be used for even more people, "including younger people in whom heart disease has yet to get a start" (1). This is a good example of how a very poorly designed study showing very little (if any) benefit associated with statins, is translated into very misleading information given to the general public.

The context in which these results were presented in the *New England Journal of Medicine* is an example of how the pharmaceutical industry is sabotaging the scientific process. The WOSCOPS follow up did not tell us anything new about statins and the way the trial was conducted raises questions about the validity of any conclusions that are drawn. Yet the results were allowed to be published to show statins in a highly favourable light.

CHAPTER 14

Cholesterol-Lowering Margarines

Since the late-1990s a range of cholesterol lowering foods have appeared in supermarkets around the world. In the UK, these products come in the form of yogurt drinks and margarine spreads, however the range may be extended in the future to include other foods. The active ingredients in these products are *plant sterols*, which are said to lower cholesterol in the body by blocking the absorption of cholesterol in the gut.

A substantial global market has developed for foods that contain plant sterols. In the UK, popular brands include *Flora pro.activ* and *Benecol®*. These products are a good example of how a processed denatured food with no nutritional value can be successfully marketed to the general public as a healthy alternative.

Flora pro.activ was launched in 2000, and was backed up by a £10 million marketing campaign. In 2008, the company that owns the brand (Unilever) said it was worth £60 million in the UK alone (1). Globally, sales for products within the Flora pro.active range were £431 million in 2007. Global sales for Benecol® during the same year were £156 million (2). Other reports have quoted European sales of these products to be in the region of £500 million each year (3). Overall, US$1 billion would represent a conservative estimate of the size of the market for 'food' products that contain plant sterols.

Despite the health claims that are made about these new cholesterol-lowering foods, there are a number of very important points that must be considered before we decide to put them in to our bodies. There are some important facts that have not been communicated to the general public. The purpose of this chapter is to provide the reader with this information in order that an informed choice about them can be made. For the discussion, we specifically look at margarines and spreads. However, the information about plant sterols can be applied to any product that contains them.

What is Margarine?

Companies that make margarines and other spreads tell us that their products are a healthy alternative to butter and other traditional natural foods.

Margarines are made from vegetable oils such as sunflower oil, rapeseed oil or canola oil. These oils are obtained by mechanically pressing the relevant seeds. The processing of the seeds into oil involves a complex sequence of operations, which includes fully refining and deodorizing (4). This processing means that the finished product has been heated to a high temperature and has been exposed to various chemicals. These refined oils lose a large proportion of their nutrients during processing. This applies not only to the oils that go on to become margarines, but in fact, to all vegetable oils, with the exception of extra virgin olive oil.

The use of these refined oils means that the production of margarine gets off to a bad start. Unfortunately, as processing continues, the situation gets worse, much worse!

The misplaced association between saturated fats and heart disease provided an opportunity for the food industry. It enabled the industry to come up with alternatives to butter that could be marketed as a 'healthier option'. However, in order to exploit this opportunity a fundamental problem had to be overcome.

Foods that contain more saturated fat (like butter) are solid at room temperature. This is due to their molecular structure and it enables them to spread easily. However, foods that contain more unsaturated fats (like vegetable oils) are liquid at room temperature. The food industry needed a product that is both low in saturated fat and solid (or spreadable) at room temperature. Within nature, no such substance exists. A food that contains mostly unsaturated fats is generally liquid at room temperature. Therefore, the food industry had to create a new type of fat. This new fat is called a *hydrogenated fat* and it has been used extensively in the manufacture of margarines and butter alternatives.

Hydrogenated fats are created by adding hydrogen molecules to the chemical structure of oils under high pressure, at very high temperature, and in the presence of nickel, aluminium or other heavy metals (5). Some experts are concerned that remnants of these metals stay in the hydrogenated fat and end up in the bodies of people who eat them - adding to the general toxic load on the body (5). Heavy metals such as these are often difficult for the body to get rid off and have been linked with a wide range of degenerative conditions. For example, aluminium has been associated with psychological disorders (5, 6).

Even if the raw material used to make margarine (the vegetable oil) had any remote resemblance to a natural food before it was hydrogenated, it certainly could not be called a natural food now. The resulting product (after being heat treated and blasted with hydrogen) is alien to the human body and the long term effects of consumption have not been fully investigated.

This process of converting vegetable oils into more solid fats is desirable for the food industry. It provides an opportunity to capitalise on the misconceptions about saturated fats, the raw materials are cheap, and the finished product can stay on the supermarket selves for several months before it decays. Unlike fresh natural butter which has to be replaced regularly.

Traditionally, the process that was used by margarine manufacturers yielded a product that contained large amounts of *trans fats*. During recent years, this type of fat has received a great deal of attention. It is now well known that the trans fats found in margarines are extremely toxic to the human body and pose significant health risks. Trans fats cause heart disease: they cause inflammation and damage the endothelial cells that line the inside wall of the arteries (7).

It is ironic that for years the margarine manufacturers were promoting their products as 'heart healthy' and all the time, these products contained substantial amounts of highly toxic trans fats. Consumer awareness of trans fats has grown rapidly and since 2006 food manufacturers in America have been required to display on the labelling the amount of trans fats in their products (7).

The increased awareness of trans fats and new labelling requirements has forced manufacturers to reduce the amount of trans fats in margarine. These companies do not go into too much detail about how this has been achieved, but simply say that it is done by a "combination of full hydrogenation, fractionation and rearrangement of the fatty acids on the triglycerides" (8). This does not sound as if the product has become any more natural!

The food industry in general has benefited a great deal from the misconception that saturated fat is unhealthy, and they have vested interests in keeping the general public misinformed about this. As discussed in chapter 1, each of the different types of dietary fats has their own properties, and a balance or mix of different fatty acids is needed in order to meet the biological needs of the human body. If butter really is that bad, how on earth did the human race survive during the thousands of years before hydrogenation, oil refining, fractionation and fatty acid rearrangement processes had been developed?

Readers will recall from chapter 12 that the size of the LDL particles within the body has a profound influence on the risk for heart disease. Smaller LDL particles presenting a greater risk for heart disease and larger LDLs being associated with a longer life. Readers will also recall that dietary saturated fats actually increase the size of LDL particles. In particular, it is the saturated fatty acids that are found in butter that have this beneficial effect (9). This is something that the marketing department of margarine manufacturers are not keen to tell people about.

Plant Sterols

Plant sterols are substances that are quite similar to cholesterol. They naturally occur in plants and can be thought of as the plant equivalent of cholesterol. Both plants and humans need sterols for the membranes of every cell. Plants use plant sterols for this purpose, where as humans need cholesterol. Under normal conditions humans do not retain plant sterols. The body has an exquisite mechanism for identifying them so that only cholesterol is absorbed (10).

No one knows for sure how plant sterols reduce cholesterol levels, but it is believed that when they enter the digestive system they compete with cholesterol for spaces in the intestinal wall. Plant sterols may effectively block some of the cholesterol from being absorbed. This may have the effect of slightly reducing the level of LDLs (so called 'bad' cholesterol) in the blood.

Most people already consume a small amount of plant sterols in their normal diet. For the average diet in the UK, this amounts to around 0.25 grams per day (11). However, in order to have an effect on LDL levels, it is necessary to consume around 2 grams of plant sterols per day. This represents roughly the amount of plant sterols found in 150 apples or 425 tomatoes. Products such as Flora pro.activ and Benecol® have been formulated so that 2 grams of plant sterols can be consumed easily with normal daily use, such as spreading on bread. Clearly this level of consumption of plant sterols is not normal for the human body.

Plant sterols that are added to margarines are made from a by-product of the vegetable oil refining process or from the oil obtained from pine-wood pulp in papermaking (11, 12). The manufacturers of these products claim that they reduce LDL levels by 10-15%. Although most of the trials done on these products included only a small number of people, there are studies to show that reductions within this range are achievable (13). These reductions typically represent a lowering of LDLs by about 0.4 mmol/l. Whether this translates to any real benefit however, is another question.

The manufacturers of these cholesterol-lowering foods are capitalising on the belief that reducing the level of LDLs is beneficial and will some how lead to improvements in health. Although there may be some evidence that these products can reduce LDLs slightly, there is not a thread of evidence that anyone has actually benefited from consuming them.

As we have already seen in chapter 11, LDL levels may have nothing at all to do with heart disease. LDLs have been branded a 'villain' largely because of trials that have been done on cholesterol drugs that lower LDL levels. However, any benefit associated with the use of cholesterol lowering drugs (statins) correlate more accurately with inflammatory markers. Statin trials are designed to test the effects of the drug, not to prove that cholesterol or LDLs form a risk factor for heart disease. Focussing on a perceived risk factor takes our eye off the target and there is no proof that anyone who consumes margarines containing plant sterols will be healthier as a result.

Safety

Some margarines such as Flora pro.activ, state in the small print on the bottom of the container, that it is not recommended to consume more than 3 grams of the product per day. This is the maximum daily intake that was recommended in a report published by the European Commission Scientific Committee on Food (14). This maximum level of consumption was deemed prudent because of the "possibility that high intakes might induce undesirable effects" (14).

Manufacturers state that various studies have found the products to be safe, but again, these studies only included a small number of people. One study found that the frequency of gastrointestinal complaints increased with increasing dosage. But only 21 people were included in each group, so it is impossible to draw any meaningful conclusions (15). At the very least, there is a great need for larger studies to be done to investigate these effects.

Plant Sterols Lower Nutrient Levels

Plant sterols reduce the absorption of fat soluble vitamins. This is something that is not written on the packaging of margarines and other products that contain plant sterols. Various studies have shown that the absorption of *carotenes* is reduced by up to 25% (11). Carotenes are the precursors (or raw materials) that the body uses to make vitamin A. Some studies also show that vitamin E is reduced by around 8% (11). So, even if the reduction in LDL 'cholesterol' is believed to provide some benefit, this is off-set by the reduction in the absorption of vital nutrients.

As discussed in chapter 10, carotenes and vitamin E are *antioxidants* and they may help to protect against heart disease.

Vitamin A is important for the physical development of the body: being essential for the growth of bones, teeth, muscles and other tissues. It also enhances the immune system (16). Any inflammation within the body greatly increases the demand for vitamin A (16). Readers will recall from chapter 11 that heart disease is mostly an inflammatory condition. Therefore, if plant sterols can potentially lower vitamin A levels, they should be avoided. Butter on the other hand provides one of the best sources of vitamin A (16).

Manufacturers of margarines containing plant sterols are fully aware of the fact that their products reduce levels of certain vitamins within the body. Scientists who work for these companies suggest that more fruit and vegetables should be eaten in order to compensate for the loss of nutrients associated with these products (17). This simply confirms that plant sterols are not meant to be consumed in such concentrated forms.

The European Commission recommended that consumers are made aware of the fact that plant sterols can lower vitamin levels (14). However, no effort has been made to inform consumers about this. Perhaps manufacturers are worried this knowledge, combined with the fact that these products are expensive, may deter consumers from buying plant sterol products?

Omega 3 and Margarine

Some manufacturers of margarines have been keen to advertise the fact that their product contains omega 3 fatty acids. Readers will recall from chapter 1 that omega 3 is one of the *essential fatty acids*. Several sources of information suggest that human beings evolved on a diet that contained roughly equal proportions of omega 3 and omega 6 essential fatty acids (18). Western diets contain too much omega 6. This is due to a number of factors including the over-consumption of grain based foods and vegetable oils that contain large amounts of omega 6. This imbalance of omega 6 to omega 3 is associated with an increased risk for developing heart disease and other serious conditions (18).

Some margarines do contain omega 3, but they also contain much more omega 6. The labels on these products reveal that they contain five or six times more omega 6 than omega 3 (depending on the specific product that is chosen). Consuming margarine will only contribute to the existing imbalance of essential fatty acids that most people in the industrialised world already have. Hence, contradicting the 'heart healthy' image that the margarine industry has spent millions of pounds trying to portray. Incidentally, natural butter contains roughly equal amounts of omega 3 and omega 6 (19).

Quick Reference Guide to Natural Food

In chapter 4 the need to eat food in its *natural* state was emphasised as the first law of nutrition. This means that all processed and *de-natured* food should be avoided as much as possible. De-natured food simply refers to food that has been made less natural through processing or the addition of additives. This section provides a basic description of what types of foods should generally be avoided and which should be included in the diet. The intention is not by any means to provide a detailed diet plan, but simply to provide a basic description of what is generally meant by *natural food*.

Foods to **avoid** include:

✗ Commercially produced (factory farmed) non-organic meats
✗ Commercially produced (factory farmed) non-organic poultry
✗ Farmed fish and other seafood
✗ Soy bean products including tofu, soy milk
✗ Semi-skimmed and skimmed milk
✗ 'Ready' meals and other processed foods
✗ Foods containing artificial colours, preservatives, flavours
✗ Foods containing sodium nitrite and potassium nitrate
✗ Foods containing hydrogenated fats or oils and *trans fats*
✗ Tinned/canned fruit and vegetables

✗   Roasted or salted nuts
✗   Refined grain based foods (white bread, white rice, white flour etc)
✗   All vegetable oils except olive oil
✗   All margarines
✗   Table salt
✗   Tap water
✗   All sugary drinks
✗   Sparkling/fizzy water
✗   Sweets
✗   Cakes and biscuits (commercially produced)
✗   All artificial sweeteners
✗   Powdered milk
✗   Most protein drinks/milkshakes (very few of them are fit for consumption)
✗   Multi-vitamin and multi-mineral supplements (especially synthetic forms)

Natural foods and drinks to **include** in your diet:

✓   Organic meats such as: beef, lamb, pork, liver and other organ meats, buffalo, venison and other game meats
✓   Cured meat (but not those containing sodium nitrite or potassium nitrate)
✓   Smoked fish
✓   Organic or free range poultry such as: chicken and turkey
✓   Fish and other seafood (not farmed)
✓   Organic and free range eggs
✓   Beans/legumes
✓   Fresh or frozen vegetables (ideally locally produced and organic)
✓   Freshly prepared vegetable juices

- ✓ Homemade soups
- ✓ Small to moderate amounts of fresh fruit (ideally locally produced and organic)
- ✓ Small to moderate amounts of miso soup and soy sauce
- ✓ Small to moderate amounts of whole milk (ideally unpasturised and organic)
- ✓ Cheese (ideally unpasturised and/or organic)
- ✓ Moderate amounts of nuts and whole seeds
- ✓ Absolute minimal amount of whole grain based foods (wholemeal bread, rye bread, oats, brown rice, etc)
- ✓ Butter
- ✓ Ghee (clarified butter)
- ✓ Lard
- ✓ Duck fat and goose fat
- ✓ Coconut oil
- ✓ Virgin olive oil
- ✓ Fresh herbs and spices
- ✓ Organic coffee (1 or 2 cups per day)
- ✓ Herbal teas
- ✓ Filtered water
- ✓ Bottled still mineral water (glass bottles are best)
- ✓ Only the best quality sea salt (e.g. Celtic Salt)
- ✓ Only use vitamin and mineral supplements based on your *Metabolic Type* (visit www.29billion.com for information)

Food Preparation

Avoid microwave food of all kinds and avoid cooking with aluminium pots, pans and aluminium foil. Also minimise fried food. Do use stainless steel, cast iron, glass and un-chipped enamel cookware.

Your Individuality

The second law of nutrition (which is equally as important as the first law) states that nutrition must be based on the individual person. A healthy food for one person may not be healthy for someone else.

The quantity of protein, fat and carbohydrate that we should aim for really does depend on our individual metabolism and the way that we as individuals process foods.

Generally, proteins consist of meat, poultry, fish, other seafood and eggs. Each of us should aim for at least three serving of protein each day. The size of each of the servings depends on our Metabolic Type (visit www.29billion.com for more information).

Metabolic Typing™ also determines the specific foods that will help to balance metabolism. This has far reaching effects and provides an excellent opportunity to improve health and reach our ideal weight.

REFERENCES

Chapter 1

1. Wharton, CH 2001 "Metabolic Man: Ten Thousand Years from Eden" WinMark Publishing, Orlando, Florida
2. Hayden, B 1981 "Subsistence and Ecological Adaptations of Modern Hunter-Gatherers" In "Omnivorous Primates" Edited by Harding, R and Teleki, G. Columbia University Press, New York
3. Fallon, S and Enig, MG 1999 "Caveman Cuisine" Published online by the Weston A. Price Foundation. Available at; http://www.westonaprice.org/traditional_diets/caveman_cuisine.html (Accessed May 18, 2008)
4. Stefansson, V 2004 "My Life with the Eskimo" Kessinger Publishing
5. Ash, M and Kane, E "Fatty Acids: The Last Nutritional Frontier" Published in CAM Magazine April 2005. Available at; http://www.nutri-linkltd.co.uk/documents/FattyAcidsthenextfrontierVs2.pdf (Accessed May 19, 2008)
6. Broadhurst, CL "Balanced Intakes of Natural Triglycerides for Optimum Nutrition: An Evolutionary and Phytochemical Perspective" Medical Hypothesis 1997; 49:247-261
7. Fallon, S and Enig, M. 2001 "Nourishing Traditions: The Cookbook that Challenges politically Correct Nutrition and the Diet Dictocrats" NewTrends, Washington DC
8. Campbell-McBride, N 2004 "Gut and Psychology Syndrome" Mediform Publishing, Cambridge, UK
9. Brisson, GJ 1981 "Lipids in Human Nutrition: An Appraisal of Some Dietary Concepts" Jack Burgess, New Jersey
10. Thies, F et al. "Association of n-3 Polyunsaturated Fatty Acids with Stability of Atherosclerotic Plaques: A Random Controlled Trial" Lancet 2003; 361:477-485
11. Smith, RL 1993 "The Cholesterol Conspiracy" Warren Green, Missouri
12. Simopoulos, AP "The Importance of the Ratio of Omega-6/Omega-3 Essential Fatty Acids" Biomedicine and Pharmacotherapy 2002; 56:365-379

Chapter 2

1. Ford, ES et al. "Explaining the Decrease in U.S. Deaths from Coronary Disease, 1980–2000" New England Journal of Medicine 2007; 356:2388-2398

2. "Mortality" Chapter 1 of the British Heart Foundation Coronary Heart Disease Statistics. July 2007 Available at: http://www.heartstats.org/datapage .asp?id=6799 (Accessed 10 February 2008)

3. Unal, B, Critchley, JA, and Capewell, S "Explaining the Decline in Coronary Heart Disease Mortality in England and Wales Between 1981 and 2000" Circulation 2004; 109:1101-1107

4. "Morbidity" Chapter 2 of the British Heart Foundation Coronary Heart Disease Statistics. July 2007 Available at: http://www.heartstats.org/ datapage.asp?id=6799

5. "Diabetes" Chapter 12 of the British Heart Foundation Coronary Heart Disease Statistics. July 2007 Available at: http://www.heartstats.org/datapage .asp?id=6799

6. The National Diet and Nutrition Survey: Adults Aged 19 to 64 Years, 2003. An Office for National Statistics Publication. Available at: http://www.statistics.gov.uk/ ssd/surveys/national_diet_nutrition_survey_adults.asp (Accessed on 19 December 2007)

7. "Prevalence of Risk Factors for CVD in People with Diabetes" Chapter 4 of the British Heart Foundation Coronary Heart Disease Statistics: Diabetes Supplement. November 2001 Available at: http://www.heartstats.org/ datapage.asp?id=711 (Accessed 10 February 2008)

8. Zaninotto, P et al. "Forecasting Obesity to 2010" Table 6. July 2006. Royal Free and University College Medical School.

9. British Nutrition Foundation "Nutrient Requirements and Recommendations" Available at: http://www.nutrition.org.uk/home.asp?siteId=43&sectionId =414&subSectionId=320&parentSection=299&which=1#1008 (Accessed on 9 January 2008)

10. British Nutrition Foundation "Energy" Available at: http:// www.nutrition.org.uk/home.asp?siteId=43&sectionId=606&subSubSectionId=3 24&subSectionId=320&parentSection=299&which=1 (Accessed February 26, 2008)

11. Scientific Advisory Committee on Nutrition (SACN) Annual Report 2006. Available at; http://www.sacn.gov.uk/reports/ (Accessed May 22, 2008)

12. British Nutrition Foundation "About BNF" Available at: http:// www.nutrition.org.uk/home.asp?siteId=43&sectionId=305&which=7 (Accessed on 9 January 2008)

13. British Nutrition Foundation "BNF Member Companies" Available at: http://www.nutrition.org.uk/home.asp?siteId=43&sectionId=352&parentSectio n=305&which=7 (Accessed on 9 January 2008)

14. The British Nutrition Foundation "Financial Statements for the Year Ended 31st May 2006" Available at: http://www.nutrition.org.uk/home.asp?siteId =43&sectionId=735&parentSection=305&which=7 (Accessed 11 January 2008)

Chapter 3

1. British Nutrition Foundation "The Eatwell Plate" Available at: http://www.nutrition.org.uk/home.asp?siteId=43&sectionId=874&subSectionId=320&parentSection=299&which=1 (Accessed February 28, 2008)
2. British Nutrition Foundation "Energy" Available at: http://www.nutrition.org.uk/home.asp?siteId=43&sectionId=606&subSubSectionId=324&subSectionId=320&parentSection=299&which=1 (Accessed February 26, 2008)
3. Bray, J and Hoggan, R 2002 "Dangerous Grains" Avery, New York
4. Catassi, C "Where Is Celiac Disease Coming From and Why?" Journal of Pediatric Gastroenterology and Nutrition 2005; 40:279-282
5. Brehm, B et al. "A Randomized Trial Comparing a Very Low Carbohydrate Diet and a Calorie-Restricted Low Fat Diet on Body Weight and Cardiovascular Risk Factors in Healthy Women" Journal of Clinical Endocrinology and Metabolism 2003; 88(4):1617-1623
6. Brand, JC et al. "Low-Glycemic Index Foods Improve Long-Term Glycemic Control in NIDDM" Diabetes Care 1991; 14:95-101
7. Gannon, MC and Nuttall, FQ "Effect of a High-Protein, Low-Carbohydrate Diet on Blood Glucose Control in People With Type 2 Diabetes" Diabetes 2004; 53:2375-2382
8. Gallop, R 2005 "The GI Diet: The Easy, Healthy Way to Permanent Weight Loss" Virgin Books
9. Chek, P 2004 "How to Eat, Move and Be Healthy" Chek Publications, San Diego
10. Robinson, J 2004 "Pasture Perfect: The Far Reaching Effects of Choosing Meat, Eggs, and Dairy Products from Grass-Fed Animals" Vashon Island Press, Washington
11. Ludwig, DS "The Glycemic Index: Physiological Mechanisms Relating to Obesity, Diabetes, and Cardiovascular Disease" Journal of the American Medical Association 2002; 287:2414-2423
12. Hu, FB et al. "Trends in the Incidence of Coronary Heart Disease and Changes in Diet and Lifestyle in Women" New England Journal of Medicine 2000; 343:530-537
13. Gardner, CD et al. "Comparison of the Atkins, Zone, Ornish and LEARN Diets for Change in Weight and Related Risk Factors among Overweight Premenopausal Women". Journal of the American Medical Association 2007; 297:969-977
14. Yancy, WS et al. "A Low-Carbohydrate, Ketogenic Diet Verses a Low-Fat Diet to Treat Obesity and Hyperlipidemia". Annals of Internal Medicine 2004; 140:769-777
15. Foster, GD et al. "A Randomized Trial of a Low-Carbohydrate Diet for Obesity" New England Journal of Medicine 2003; 348:2082-2090

16. Brehm, BJ et al. "A Randomized Trial Comparing a Very Low Carbohydrate Diet and a Calorie-Restricted Low Fat Diet on Body Weight and Cardiovascular Risk Factors in Healthy Women". The Journal of Clinical Endocrinology and Metabolism 2003; 88(4):1617-1623

17. Stern, L et al. "The Effects of Low-Carbohydrate Verses Conventional Weight Loss Diets in Severely Obese Adults: One-Year Follow-up of a Randomized Trial". Annals of Internal Medicine 2004; 140:778-785

18. Samaha, FF et al. "A Low-Carbohydrate as Compared with a Low-Fat Diet in Severe Obesity" New England Journal of Medicine 2003; 348:2074-2081

19. Shai, I et al. "Weight Loss with a Low-Carbohydrate, Mediterranean, or Low-Fat Diet" New England Journal of Medicine 2008; 359:229-241

20. Allan, CB and Lutz, W, 2000 "Life Without Bread: How a Low-Carbohydrate Diet Can Save Your Life" McGraw Hill, New York

21. Shallenberger, F, 2006 "The Type 2 Diabetes Breakthrough: A Revolutionary Approach to Treating Type 2 Diabetes" Basic Health Publications, California

22. "Cholesterol" British Heart Foundation Website Page. Available at: http://www.bhf.org.uk/keeping_your_heart_healthy/preventing_heart_disease/cholesterol.aspx (Accessed March 7, 2008)

23. "Triglycerides" Factsheet Published by HEART UK. Available at: http://www.heartuk.org.uk/new/pages/info/sheets.html (Accessed March 7, 2008)

24. Liu, S et al. "Dietary Glycemic Load assessed by Food-Frequency Questionnaire in Relation to Plasma High-Density-Lipoprotein Cholesterol and Fasting Plasma Triacylglycerols in Postmenopausal Women" American Journal of Clinical Nutrition 2001;73:560-566

25. Radhika, G et al. "Dietary Carbohydrates, Glycemic Load and Serum High-Density Lipoprotein Cholesterol Concentrations Among South Indian Adults" European Journal of Clinical Nutrition. Advance Online Publication November 7, 2007

26. Garg, A, Grundy, SM and Koffler, M "Effect of High Carbohydrate Intake on Hyperglycemia, Islet Function, and Plasma Lipoproteins in NIDDM" Diabetes Care 1992; 15:1572-1580

27. Garg, A et al. "Effects of Varying Carbohydrate Content of Diet in Patients with Non-Insulin-Dependent Diabetes Mellitus" Journal of the American Medical Association 1994; 271:1421-1428

28. Appel. LJ et al. "Effects of Protein, Monounsaturated Fat, and Carbohydrate Intake on Blood Pressure and Serum Lipids" Journal of the American Medical Association 2005; 294: 2455-2464

29. Mozaffarian, D, Rimm, EB, and Herrington, DM "Dietary Fats, Carbohydrate, and Progression of Coronary Atherosclerosis in Postmenopausal Women" American Journal of Clinical Nutrition 2004; 80(5):1175-1184

30. Dunder, K et al. "Increase in Blood Glucose Concentration during Antihypertensive Treatment as a Predictor of Myocardial Infarction: Population Based Cohort Study" British Medical Journal 2003; 326:681-685

31. Saydah, SH et al. "Postchallenge Hyperglycemia and Mortality in a National Sample of U.S. Adults" Diabetes Care 2001; 24:1397-1402

32. Qiao, Q et al. "Two Prospective Studies found that Elevated 2-hr Glucose Predicted Male Mortality Independent of Fasting Glucose and HbA1c" Journal of Clinical Epidemiology 2004; 57:590-596

33. Temelkova-Kurktschiev, TS et al. "Postchallenge Plasma Glucose and Glycemic Spikes Are More Strongly Associated with Atherosclerosis than Fasting Glucose or HbA1c Level" Diabetes Care 2000; 23:1830-1834

34. Balkau, B et al. "High Blood Glucose Concentration is a Risk Factor for Mortality in Middle-Aged Nondiabetic Men. 20-year Follow-Up in the Whitehall Study, the Paris Prospective Study, and the Helsinki Policemen Study" Diabetes Care 1998; 21:360-367

35. Liu, S et al. "A Prospective Study of Dietary Glycemic Load, Carbohydrate Intake, and Risk of Coronary Heart Disease in US Women" American Journal of Clinical Nutrition 2000; 71:1455-1461

36. Levitan, EB et al. "Is Nondiabetic Hyperglycemia a Risk Factor for Cardiovascular Disease? A Meta-analysis of Prospective Studies" Archives of Internal Medicine 2004; 164:2147-2155

37. Danaei, G et al. "Global and Regional Mortality from Ischaemic Heart Disease and Stroke Attributable to Higher-Than-Optimum Blood Glucose Concentration: Comparative Risk Assessment" Lancet 2006; 368:1651-1659

38. Wei, M et al. "Effects of Diabetes and Level of Glycemia on All-Cause and Cardiovascular Mortality. The San Antonio Heart Study" Diabetes Care 1998; 21:1167-1172

39. Rodriguez, BL et al. "Glucose Intolerance and 23-Year Risk of Coronary Heart Disease and Total Mortality: The Honolulu Heart Program" Diabetes Care 1999; 22:1262-1265

40. Vaccaro, O, Ruth, KJ, and Stamler, J "Relationship of Postload Plasma Glucose to Mortality with 19-yr Follow-Up. Comparison of One versus Two Plasma Glucose Measurements in the Chicago Peoples Gas Company Study" Diabetes Care 1992; 15:1328-1334

41. Lowe, LP et al. "Diabetes, Asymptomatic Hyperglycemia, and 22-Year Mortality in Black and White Men. The Chicago Heart Association Detection Project in Industry Study" Diabetes Care 1997; 20:163-169

42. Campbell-McBride, N 2004 "Gut and Psychology Syndrome" Mediform Publishing, Cambridge, UK

43. Schroeder, HA 1973 "The Trace Elements and Man: Some Positive and Negative Aspects" Devin-Adair, Greenwich, Connecticut

44. DeCava, JA. 2006 "The Real Truth About Vitamins and Anti-oxidants" 2nd Edition Selene River Press, Fort Collins
45. Zheng, JJ et al. "Measurement of Zinc Bioavailability from Beef and a Ready-to-Eat High- Fiber Breakfast Cereal in Humans: Application of a Whole-Gut Lavage Technique" American Journal of Clinical Nutrition 1993; 58:902-907
46. Widdowson, EM and McCance, RA "Iron Exchanges of Adults on White and Brown Bread Diets" Lancet 1942; 1:588-591
47. Reinhold, JG et al. "Binding of Zinc to Fiber and Other Solids of Wholemeal Bread" in "Trace Elements in Human Health and Disease Volume 1: Zinc and Copper" Academic Press, 1976
48. Hallberg, L, Rossander, L and Skanberg, AB "Phytates and the Inhibitory Effect of Bran on Iron Absorption in Man" American Journal of Clinical Nutrition 1987; 45:988-996
49. Fallon, S and Enig, M. 2001 "Nourishing Traditions: The Cookbook that Challenges politically Correct Nutrition and the Diet Dictocrats" NewTrends, Washington DC
50. Murray, M 1999 "5-HTP: The Natural Way to Overcome Depression, Obesity, and Insomnia" Bantam Books, New York
51. Braverman, ER 2005 "The Edge Effect: Achieve Total Health and Longevity with the Balanced Brain Advantage" Sterling Publishing, New York

Chapter 4

1. Price, WA 2003 "Nutrition and Physical Degeneration" 6th Edition Price-Pottenger Nutrition Foundation (www.price-pottenger.org)
2. "To Study Eskimo Life" New York Times September 3, 1921
3. Cleave, TL 1974 "The Saccharine Disease" John Wright and Sons, Bristol
4. "American Indian/Alaska Native Profile" Published by: The Office of Minority Health. Available at: http://www.omhrc.gov/templates/browse.aspx?lvl=3&lvlid=26 (Accessed May 8, 2008)
5. "We Have the Power to Prevent Diabetes" Published by: National Diabetes Education Program. Available at: http://ndep.nih.gov/campaigns/SmallSteps/power_tips/index.htm (Accessed May 8, 2008)
6. "The Diabetes Epidemic among American Indians and Alaska Natives" Published by; National Diabetes Education Program. Available at: http://ndep.nih.gov/diabetes/pubs/FS_AmIndian.pdf (Accessed May 8, 2008)
7. "The Heart, the Drum" Video produced by the National Heart, Lung and Blood Institute. Available at: http://hp2010.nhlbihin.net/minority/nat_frameset.htm (Accessed May 8, 2008)
8. O'Dea, K "Marked Improvement in Carbohydrate and Lipid Metabolism in Diabetic Australian Aborigines after Temporary Reversion to Traditional

Lifestyle" Diabetes 1984; 33:596-603

9. Baschetti, R "Diabetes in Aboriginal Populations" Canadian Medical Association Journal 2000; 162:969

10. Kaplan, H et al. "A Theory of Human Life History Evolution: Diet, Intelligence, and Longevity" Evolutionary Anthropology 2000; 9:156-185

11. Cordain, L et al. "The Paradoxical Nature of Humter-Gatherer Diets: Meat-Based, Yet Non-Atherogenic" European Journal of Clinical Nutrition 2002; 56(Suppl 1):S42-S52

12. Williams, RJ 1998 "Biochemical Individuality: The Basis for the Genetotrophic Concept" Keats Publishing, Connecticut

13. Wolcott, W 2002 "The Metabolic Typing Diet" Broadway Books, New York

Chapter 5

1. Moore, Thomas. 1989 "Heart Failure: A Searing Report on Modern Medicine at Its Best and Worst" Touchstone, New York.

2. Smith, RL 1993 "The Cholesterol Conspiracy" Warren Green, Missouri

3. McGee, Charles. 2001 "Heart Frauds: Uncovering the Biggest Health Scam in History" HealthWise, Colorado Springs.

4. Colpo, Anthony. 2006 "The Great Cholesterol Con: Why Everything You've Told About Cholesterol, Diet and Heart Disease is Wrong!" www.Lulu.com

5. British Heart Foundation Booklet "Reducing Your Blood Cholesterol". Available at: www.bhf.org.uk (Accessed October 28, 2007)

6. Barres, BA, Smith, SJ. "Cholesterol - Making or Breaking the Synapse" Science Nov 2001; Vol. 294:1296-1297

7. Brisson, GJ 1981 "Lipids in Human Nutrition: An Appraisal of Some Dietary Concepts" Jack Burgess, New Jersey

8. "Blood Cholesterol" Chapter 10 of the British Heart Foundation Coronary Heart Disease Statistics. July 2007 Available at: http://www.heartstats.org/datapage.asp?id=6799 (Accessed on April 15, 2007)

9. Kannel, WB, Castelli, WP and Gordon, T "Cholesterol in the Prediction of Atherosclerotic Disease: New Perspectives based on the Framingham Study" Annals of Internal Medicine 1979; 90:85-91

10. British Heart Foundation Booklet "Reducing Your Blood Cholesterol". Available from www.bhf.org.uk (Accessed October 28, 2007) Please note that a check on this reference completed during August 2008 revealed that changes have been made to this booklet. The version that was referenced in October 2007 contained a diagram showing the contribution various 'risk factors' make to the risk of developing heart disease. However, this diagram has been omitted from the version that is available for download as of August 2008. The previous version containing this diagram (showing that more than half of people who die

of heart disease have low cholesterol) is available from www.29billion.com

11. Durrington, P "Dyslipidaemia" Lancet 2003; 362:717-731

12. Tonkin, AM et al. "Effects of Pravastatin in 3260 Patients with Unstable Angina: Results from the LIPID Study" Lancet 2000; 355:1871-1875

13. World Health Organisation (WHO) Global InfoBase Country Data for Australia. Available at: http://www.who.int/infobase/report.aspx?rid= 115&dm=17&iso=AUS (Accessed April 21, 2008)

14. World Health Organisation (WHO) Global InfoBase Country Data for New Zealand. Available at: http://www.who.int/infobase/report.aspx?rid= 115&iso=NZL&filterButton=Filter+Indicators&dm=17 (Accessed April 21, 2008)

15. Rubins, HB et al. "Distribution of Lipids in 8,500 Men with Coronary Artery Disease" The American Journal of Cardiology 1995; 75:1202-1205

16. World Health Organisation (WHO) Global InfoBase Country Data for United States. Available at: http://www.who.int/infobase/reportviewer.aspx? rptcode=ALL&uncode=840&dm=17&surveycode=101236a1 (Accessed April 21, 2008)

17. BBC News "1.5m More to get Cholesterol Drug" May 27, 2008 Available at: http://news.bbc.co.uk/1/hi/health/7421731.stm (Accessed May 28, 2008)

18. The National Diet and Nutrition Survey: Adults Aged 19 to 64 Years 2003. Vol. 5. An Office for National Statistics Publication. Available at: http://www.statistics.gov.uk/statbase/Product.asp?vlnk=9761&More=N (Accessed 19 November 2007)

19. British Heart Foundation "All About Statins" Available at: http:// www.bhf.org.uk/living_with_heart_conditions/treatment/medicines_for_the_ heart/statins.aspx (Accessed 19 November 2007)

20. Kendrick, M. 2007 "The Great Cholesterol Con: The Truth About What Really Causes Heart Disease and How to Avoid It" John Blake, London

21. Ravnskov, U 2003 "The Cholesterol Myths: Exposing the Fallacy that Cholesterol and Saturated Fat Cause Heart Disease" NewTrends, Washington, DC

22. Kaunitz, H "Cholesterol and Repair Processes in Arteriosclerosis" Lipids 1978; 13(5):373-374

23. Kaunitz, H "Dietary Lipids and Arteriosclerosis" Journal of the American Oil Chemists' Society 1975; 52(8): 293-297

Chapter 6

1. Lowering Blood Cholesterol to Prevent Heart Disease. National Institutes of Health Consensus Development Conference Statement December 10-12, 1984. Available at: http://consensus.nih.gov/1984/1984Cholesterol047html.htm (Accessed November 1, 2007)

2. Biss, K, et al. "Some Unique Biological Characteristics of the Masai of East Africa" New England Journal of Medicine 1971; Vol. 284, 13: 694-699

3. The National Diet and Nutrition Survey: Adults Aged 19 to 64 Years 2003. Vol. 2 A National Statistics Publication

4. Department of Health. Report on Health and Social Subjects: 46. Nutritional Aspects of Cardiovascular Disease. HMSO London 1994

5. Food and Agriculture Organisation. Food and Nutrition Paper: 57. Fats and Oils in Human Nutrition. FAO Rome 1994

6. Ravnskov, Uffe. 2003 "The Cholesterol Myths: Exposing the Fallacy that Cholesterol and Saturated Fat Cause Heart Disease" NewTrends, Washington, DC

7. Keys, A et al. "Lessons from Serum Cholesterol Studies in Japan, Hawaii and Los Angeles" Annals of Internal Medicine 1958; 48:83-94

8. Fallon, S and Enig, M. 2001 "Nourishing Traditions: The Cookbook that Challenges Politically Correct Nutrition and the Diet Dictocrats" NewTrends, Washington DC

9. Colpo, Anthony. 2006 "The Great Cholesterol Con: Why Everything You've Told About Cholesterol, Diet and Heart Disease is Wrong!" www.Lulu.com

10. Kendrick, M. 2007 "The Great Cholesterol Con: The Truth About What Really Causes Heart Disease and How to Avoid It" John Blake, London

11. Spady, DK, Dietschy, JM. "Interaction of Dietary Cholesterol and Triglycerides In the Regulation of Hepatic Low Density Lipoprotein Transport in the Hamster". Journal of Clinical Investigation 1988; 81:300-309

12. Barnes, BO and Galton, L 1976 "Hypothyroidism: The Unsuspected Illness" Harper and Row, New York

13. Frost, G et al. "Glycaemic Index as a Determinant of Serum HDL-Cholesterol Concentration" The Lancet 1999; 353:1045-1048

14. Foster, GD et al. "A Randomized Trial of a Low-Carbohydrate Diet for Obesity" New England Journal of Medicine 2003; 348:2082-2090

15. Atkins, RC. 1998 "Dr Atkins' New Diet Revolution" Rev Ed. Avon Books, New York

16. Shai, I et al. "Weight Loss with a Low-Carbohydrate, Mediterranean, or Low-Fat Diet" New England Journal of Medicine 2008; 359:229-241

17. Brehm, BJ et al. "A Randomized Trial Comparing a Very Low Carbohydrate Diet and a Calorie-Restricted Low Fat Diet on Body Weight and Cardiovascular Risk Factors in Healthy Women". The Journal of Clinical Endocrinology and Metabolism 2003; 88(4):1617-1623

18. Stern, L et al. "The Effects of Low-Carbohydrate Verses Conventional Weight Loss Diets in Severely Obese Adults: One-Year Follow-up of a Randomized Trial". Annals of Internal Medicine 2004; 140:778-785

19. Yancy, WS et al. "A Low-Carbohydrate, Ketogenic Diet Verses a Low-Fat Diet

to Treat Obesity and Hyperlipidemia". Annals of Internal Medicine 2004; 140:769-777
20. Gardner, CD et al. "Comparison of the Atkins, Zone, Ornish and LEARN Diets for Change in Weight and Related Risk Factors among Overweight Premenopausal Women". Journal of the American Medical Association 2007; 297:969-977
21. Liu, S et al. "A Prospective Study of Dietary Glycemic Load, Carbohydrate Intake, and Risk of Coronary Heart Disease in US Women" American Journal of Clinical Nutrition 2000; 71:1455-1461
22. Mozaffarian, D, Rimm, EB, and Herrington, DM "Dietary Fats, Carbohydrate, and Progression of Coronary Atherosclerosis in Postmenopausal Women" American Journal of Clinical Nutrition 2004; 80(5):1175-1184

Chapter 7

1. The World Health Organisation Global InfoBase. Available at: http://www.who.int/infobase/report.aspx (Accessed 27 November 2007)
2. "Health Survey for England 2003" Department of Health 2004. DH: London
3. "Blood Cholesterol" Chapter 10 of the British Heart Foundation Coronary Heart Disease Statistics. July 2007 Available at: http://www.heartstats.org/datapage.asp?id=6799
4. "Treatment" Chapter 3 of the British Heart Foundation Coronary Heart Disease Statistics. July 2007 Available at: http://www.heartstats.org/datapage.asp?id=6799
5. "Heart Health Organisations Urge Patients to Continue with Statin Treatments" Published on the British Heart Foundation Website. Available at; http://www.bhf.org.uk/default.aspx?page=8462 (Accessed 27 November 2007)
6. World Health Organisation MONICA Database: www.ktl.fi/publications/monica. The data is also available from the British Heart Foundation at www.heartstats.org
7. World Health Organisation Global InfoBase Country Comparison. Available at: http://www.who.int/infobase/comparestart.aspx (Accessed 27 November 2007)
8. Joint British Societies' Guidelines on Prevention of Cardiovascular Disease in Clinical Practice" Heart 2005; 91(suppl_5):v1-v52
9. Global Average Cholesterol can be calculated from the data contained in the World Health Organisation Global InfoBase Country Comparison. Available at: http://www.who.int/infobase/comparestart.aspx (Accessed 27 November 2007)
10. "Morbidity" Chapter 2 of the British Heart Foundation Coronary Heart Disease Statistics. July 2007 Available at: http://www.heartstats.org/

datapage.asp?id=6799

11. Krumholz, H et al. "Lack of Association Between Cholesterol and Coronary Heart Disease Mortality and Morbidity and All-Cause Mortality in Persons Older Than 70 Years" Journal of the American Medical Association 1994; 272:1335-1340

12. Weverling-Rijnsburger, AW et al. "Total Cholesterol and Risk of Mortality in the Oldest Old" Lancet 1997; 350:1119-1123

13. Krum, H and McMurray, JJ. "Statins and Chronic Heart Failure: Do We Need a Large-Scale Outcome Trial?" Journal of the American College of Cardiology 2002; 39(10):1567-1573.

14. Böhm M et al. "Heart Failure and Statins — Why Do We Need a Clinical Trial?" Zeitschrift für Kardiologie 2005; 94:223-2230.

15. Kjekshus J. "A Statin In The Treatment of Heart Failure? Controlled Rosuvastatin Multinational Study in Heart Failure (CORONA): Study Design and Baseline Characteristics" European Journal of Heart Failure 2005; 7:1059-1069.

16. Cleland, JG, et al. "Threats, Opportunities, and Statins in the Modern Management of Heart Failure" European Heart Journal 2006; 27:641-643.

17. Horwich, TB et al. "Low Serum Total Cholesterol Is Associated With Marked Increase in Mortality in Advanced Heart Failure" Journal of Cardiac Failure 2002; 8:216-224.

18. Rauchhaus, M et al. "The Relationship between Cholesterol and Survival in Patients with Chronic Heart Failure" Journal of the American College Cardiology 2003; 42:1933-1940.

19. Rauchhaus, M et al. "The Endotoxin-Lipoprotein Hypothesis" The Lancet 2000; 356(9233):930-933

20. Iribarren, C et al. "Cohort Study of Serum Total Cholesterol and In-Hospital Incidence of Infectious Diseases" Epidemiology and Infection 1998;121:335-347

21. Schatz, IJ et al. "Cholesterol and All-Cause Mortality in Elderly People From the Honolulu Heart Program: A Cohort Study" The Lancet 2001; 358:351-355

22. Huang, X et al. " Lower Low-Density Lipoprotein Cholesterol Levels Are Associated With Parkinson's Disease" Movement Disorders 2007; 22(3):377-381

23. British Heart Foundation Booklet "Reducing Your Blood Cholesterol". Available from www.bhf.org.uk (Accessed October 28, 2007) Please note that a check on this reference completed during August 2008 revealed that changes have been made to this booklet. The version that was referenced in October 2007 contained a diagram showing the contribution various 'risk factors' make to the risk of developing heart disease. However, this diagram has been omitted from the version that is available for download as of August 2008. The previous version containing this diagram (showing that more than half of people who die of heart disease have low cholesterol) is available from www.29billion.com

24. "The World Health Report 2002: Reducing Risks, Promoting Healthy Life" The World Health Organisation, Geneva 2003. Available from: http://

www.who.int/whr/2002/en/index.html
35. Khot, UN et al "Prevalence of Conventional Risk Factors in Patients With Coronary Heart Disease" Journal of the American Medical Association 2003; 290(7):898-904
26. Penelope, K et al. "Serum Cholesterol and Cognitive Performance in the Framingham Heart Study" Psychosomatic Medicine 2005; 67:24-30
27. "Prevalence of Risk Factors for CVD in People with Diabetes" Chapter 4 of the British Heart Foundation Coronary Heart Disease Statistics: Diabetes Supplement. 2001 Edition. Available at: http://www.heartstats.org/datapage.asp?id=3258
28. "Prevalence of Diabetes" Chapter 1 of the British Heart Foundation Coronary Heart Disease Statistics: Diabetes Supplement. 2001 Edition. Available at: http://www.heartstats.org/datapage.asp?id=3258

Chapter 8

1. Kendrick, M. 2007 "The Great Cholesterol Con: The Truth About What Really Causes Heart Disease and How to Avoid It" John Blake, London.
2. Rundek, T et al. "Atorvastatin Decreases the Coenzyme Q10 Level in the Blood of Patients at Risk for Cardiovascular Disease and Stroke" Archives of Neurology 2004; 61(6):889-892
3. Langsjoen, PH et al. "Treatment of Statin Adverse Effects with Supplemental Coenzyme Q10 and Statin Drug Discontinuation" Biofactors 2005; 25(1-4):147-52
4. David, C et al. "Congestive Heart Failure in the United States: Is There More Than Meets the I(CD Code)? The Corpus Christi Heart Project" Archives of Internal Medicine 2000;160:197-202
5. "Coronary Heart Disease Statistics: Heart Failure Supplement" British Heart Foundation 2002. Available at: http://www.ws3.heartstats.web.baigent.net/uploads/documents%5CHeartFailure2002.pdf (Accessed 28 November 2007)
6. "Heart Failure Fact Sheet" Centers for Disease Control and Prevention. September 2006 Available at: http://www.cdc.gov/DHDSP/library/pdfs/fs_heart_failure.pdf (Accessed 28 November 2007)
7. Ravnskov, U. "Should We Lower Cholesterol As Much As Possible?" British Medical Journal 2006; 332:1330-1332
8. Gheorghiade, M and Bonow, R. "Chronic Heart Failure in the United States: A Manifestation of Coronary Artery Disease" Circulation 1998; 97:282-289
9. Mortensen, SA et al. "Dose-Related Decrease of Serum Coenzyme Q10 During Treatment with HMG-CoA Reductase Inhibitors" Molecular Aspects of Medicine 1997; 18 Supplement 1:S137-144
10. Hanaki, Y et al. "Coenzyme Q10 and Coronary Artery Disease" Clinical

Investigator 1993; 71:S 112–115

11. Folkers, K et al. "Lovastatin Decreases Coenzyme Q Levels in Humans" Proceedings of the National Academy of Sciences 1990; 87:8931-8934

12. "Treatment" Chapter 3 of the British Heart Foundation Coronary Heart Disease Statistics. July 2007 Available at: http://www.heartstats.org/datapage.asp?id=6799 (Accessed 1 December 2007)

13. Hawkes, N. "The Pill of Life That Keeps On Working" The Times Newspaper. October 11 2007.

14. Hope, J. "More Women Should Be Prescribed Statins" Daily Mail Newspaper. May 11 2007. Available at: http://www.dailymail.co.uk/pages/live/articles/health/healthmain.html?in_article_id=453999&in_page_id=1774 (Accessed 28 November 2007)

15. The National Institute for Health and Clinical Excellence. "Cardiovascular Disease - statins: Guidance" January 2006. Available at: http://www.nice.org.uk/guidance/index.jsp?action=download&o=33151 (Accessed 28 November 2007)

16. Moon, J. Bogle, R. "Switching Statins" British Medical Journal 2006; 332:1344-1345.

17. Vadon, R "NHS Bill for Statins 'Could Soar' BBC News April 2, 2008 Available at: http://news.bbc.co.uk/1/hi/health/7326870.stm (Accessed April 4, 2008)

18. BBC Radio 4 Program "The Investigator" April 3, 2008 20:00hrs GMT

19. British Heart Foundation "All About Statins" Available at: http://www.bhf.org.uk/living_with_heart_conditions/treatment/medicines_for_the_heart/statins.aspx (Accessed on 28 November 2007)

20. "Blood Cholesterol" Chapter 10 of the British Heart Foundation Coronary Heart Disease Statistics. July 2007 Available at: http://www.heartstats.org/datapage.asp?id=6799 (Accessed July 1, 2008)

21. Kingsland, J. "Statins: Wonder Drugs for the Masses?" New Scientist October 2006.

22. Abramson, J and Wright, J. "Are lipid-Lowering Guidelines Evidence-Based" Lancet 2007; 369:168-169

23. Wheldon, J. "Statins Won't Prevent Women Getting Heart Disease, Claim Doctors". Daily Mail Newspaper, 23 January 2007. Available at: http://www.dailymail.co.uk/pages/live/articles/health/healthmain.html?in_article_id=430928&in_page_id=1774 (Accessed 1 December 2007)

24. Walsh, JM and Pignone, M. "Drug Treatment of Hyperlipidemia in Women" Journal of the American Medical Association 2004; 291:2243-2252

25. Isles, CG et al. "Relation Between Coronary Risk and Coronary Mortality in Women of the Renfrew and Paisley Survey: Comparison with Men" Lancet 1992; 339:702-706

26. Kjekshus, J et al. "Rosuvastatin in Older Patients with Systolic Heart Failure"

New England Journal of Medicine 2007; 357.

27. British Heart Foundation Booklet "Medicines for the Heart" 2004. Available at: http://www.bhf.org.uk/living_with_heart_conditions/treatment/medicines _for_the_heart.aspx (Accessed 3 December 2007)

28. Heart Protection Study Collaborative. "Lifetime Cost Effectiveness of Simvastatin in a Range of Risk Groups and Age Groups Derived From a Randomised Trial of 20 536 People" British Medical Journal 2006; 333:1145

29. Parker, T "Cholesterol Screening Is Urged for Young" The New York Times July 7, 2008 Available at: http://www.nytimes.com/2008/07/07/health/ 07cholesterol.html?_r=1&adxnnl=1&ref=health&adxnnlx=1218726235- mCrOPQMon+2bukc/YBWi5w&oref=slogin (Accessed August 14, 2008)

30. Boseley, S "Heart Disease: US Doctors Back Statins for 8-Year-Olds" Guardian Newspaper July 9 2008 Available at: http://www.guardian.co.uk/society/2008/ jul/09/health.medicalresearch (Accessed August 14, 2008)

31. Hope, J. "More Women Should Be Prescribed Statins" Daily Mail Newspaper, 11 May 2007. Available at: http://www.dailymail.co.uk/pages/live/ articles/health/healthmain.html?in_article_id=453999&in_page_id=1774 (Accessed 1 December 2007)

32. Kendrick, M. "Should Women be Offered Cholesterol Lowering Drugs to Prevent Cardiovascular Disease? No" British Medical Journal 2007; 334:983

33. Carey, J "Do Cholesterol Drugs Do Any Good?" BusinessWeek Magazine January 17, 2008 Available at: http://www.businessweek.com/magazine/ content/08_04/b4068052092994.htm (Accessed April 3, 2008)

34. Pfizer Inc. 2006 Financial Report. Available at: http://www.pfizer.com/ investors/financial_reports/financial_reports.jsp (Accessed 1 December 2007)

35. Smith, CC et al. "Screening for Statin-Related Toxicity: The Yield of Transaminase and Creatine Kinase Measurements In a Primary Care Setting" Archives of Internal Medicine 2003; 163:688–692

36. Ajani, UA and Ford, ES. "Has the Risk for Coronary Heart Disease Changed Among U.S. Adults?" Journal of the American College of Cardiology 2006; 48: 1177-1182

37. Barter, PJ et al. "Effects of Torcetrapib in Patients at High Risk for Coronary Events" New England Journal of Medicine 2007; 357:2109-2122

38. Rader, DJ. "Illuminating HDL – Is It Still a Viable Therapeutic Target?" New England Journal of Medicine 2007; 357:2180

39. Cutler, DM. "The Demise of the Blockbuster?" New England Journal of Medicine 2007; 356:1292-1293

Chapter 9

1. Office for National Statistics "Prescriptions Dispensed in the Community,

REFERENCES

Statistics for 1996 to 2006: England." Table 1. Available at: http://www.ic.nhs.uk/statistics-and-data-collections/primary-care/prescriptions/prescriptions-dispensed-in-the-community-1996-2006-%5Bns%5D (Accessed 28 January 2008)

2. Smith, R 2006 "The Trouble with Medical Journals" Royal Society of Medicine Press Ltd., London

3. Moynihan, R, Heath, I and Henry, D "Selling Sickness: The Pharmaceutical Industry and Disease Mongering" British Medical Journal 2002; 324:886-891

4. Mintzes, B "Disease Mongering in Drug Promotion: Do Governments Have a Regulatory Role?" PLoS Medicine 2006; 3:0461-0465

5. Heath, I "Combating Disease Mongering: Daunting but Nonetheless Essential" PLoS Medicine 2006; 3:0448-0451

6. Primatesta, P and Poulter, NR "Lipid Concentrations and the Use of Lipid Lowering Drugs: Evidence From a National Cross Sectional Survey" British Medical Journal 2000; 321:1322-1325

7. Bruckert, E "Epidemiology of Low HDL-Cholesterol: Results of Studies and Surveys" European Heart Journal 2006; 8(Supplement F):F17-F22

8. Campbell, EG et al. "A National Survey of Physician-Industry Relationships" New England Journal of Medicine 2007; 356:1742-1750

9. Campbell, EG "Doctors and Drug Companies – Scrutinizing Influential Relationships" New England Journal of Medicine 2007; 357:1796-1797

10. Wazana, A "Physicians and the Pharmaceutical Industry: Is a Gift Ever Just a Gift?" Journal of the American Medical Association 2000; 283:373-380

11. Deveugele, M et al. "Consultation Length in General Practice: Cross Sectional Study in Six European Countries" British Medical Journal 2002; 325:472-477

12. Lexchin, J et al. "Pharmaceutical Industry Sponsorship and Research Outcome and Quality: Systematic Review" British Medical Journal 2003; 326:1167-1170

13. Sterne, JAC, Egger, M and Smith, GD "Systematic Reviews in Health Care: Investigating and Dealing with Publication and Other Biases in Meta-analysis" British Medical Journal 2001; 323:101-105

14. Berenson, A "Study Reveals Doubt on Drug for Cholesterol" New York Times January 18, 2008. Available at: http://www.nytimes.com/2008/01/15/business/15drug.html?_r=1&oref=slogin (Accessed February 19, 2008)

15. Product News – "Merck/Schering-Plough Pharmaceuticals Provides Results of the ENHANCE Trial" Available at: http://www.merck.com/newsroom/press_releases/product/2008_0114.html (Accessed February 19, 2008)

16. Berenson, A "Data about Zetia Risks Was Not Fully Revealed" New York Times December 21, 2007. Available at: http://www.nytimes.com/2007/12/21/business/21drug.html?_r=1&oref=slogin (Accessed February 19, 2008)

17. Burne, J "The NHS Has Spent £74 Million On a New Heart Pill That The Makers Knew Didn't Work. How Could This Happen?" Daily Mail Newspaper.

February 14, 2008 Available at: http://www.mailonsunday.co.uk/pages/live/articles/health/healthmain.html?in_article_id=513729&in_page_id=1774 (Accessed February 19, 2008)

18. Goldacre, B "Clinical Trials and Playing by the Rules" Guardian Newspaper. January 5, 2008. Available at: http://www.guardian.co.uk/commentisfree/2008/jan/05/1 (Accessed February 19, 2008)

19. Rossebo, AB et al. "Intensive Lipid Lowering with Simvastatin and Ezetimibe in Aortic Stenosis" New England Journal of Medicine, Published at www.nejm.org September 2, 2008 (10.1056/NEJMoa0804602)

20. Peto, R et al. "Analyses of Cancer Data from Three Ezetimibe Trials" New England Journal of Medicine, Published at www.nejm.org September 2, 2008 (10.1056/NEJMsa0806603)

21. Drazen, JM et al. "Ezetimibe and Cancer — An Uncertain Association" New England Journal of Medicine, Published at www.nejm.org September 2, 2008 (10.1056/NEJMe0807200)

22. Berenson, A "Cholesterol as a Danger Has Skeptics" New York Times. January 17, 2008. Available at: http://query.nytimes.com/gst/fullpage.html?res=9A01E0D6133FF934A25752C0A96E9C8B63&sec=&spon=&pagewanted=2 (Accessed February 19, 2008)

23. Turner, EH "Selective Publication of Antidepressant Trials and Its Influence on Apparent Efficacy" New England Journal of Medicine 2008; 358:252-260

24. Kirsch, I et al. "Initial Severity and Antidepressant Benefits: A Meta-Analysis of Data Submitted to the Food and Drug Administration" PLoS Medicine 2008; 5:0260-0268

25. Boseley, S "Prozac, Used by 40m People, Does Not Work Say Scientists" Guardian Newspaper. February 26, 2008. Available at: http://www.guardian.co.uk/society/2008/feb/26/mentalhealth.medicalresearch (Accessed February 26, 2008)

26. Schwitzer, G et al. "What Are the Roles and Responsibilities of the Media in Disseminating Health Information?" PLoS Medicine 2005; 2:0576-0582

27. Barriaux, M "Glaxo Chief Curses Media and Issues Profit Warning" Guardian February 8, 2008. Available at: http://www.guardian.co.uk/business/2008/feb/08/glaxosmithklinebusiness.pharmaceuticals (Accessed February 19, 2008)

28. Nissen, SE and Wolski, K "Effect of Rosiglitazone on the Risk of Myocardial Infarction and Death from Cardiovascular Causes" New England Journal of Medicine 2007; 356:2457-2471

29. Foley, S "GSK Shares Slump after Diabetes Drug is linked to Heart Attacks" The Independent May 22, 2007. Available at: http://www.independent.co.uk/news/business/news/gsk-shares-slump-after-diabetes-drug-is-linked-to-heart-attacks-449874.html (Accessed February 19, 2008)

30. Laurance, J "Leading Diabetes Drug 'Raises Risk of Heart Attack'" The

Independent May 22, 2007. Available at: http://www.independent.co.uk/ life-style/health-and-wellbeing/health-news/leading-diabetes-drug-raises-risk-of-h eart-attack-449861.html (Accessed February 19, 2008)

31. Foley, S "Is Avandia set to be Glaxo's Vioxx?" The Independent June 6, 2007. Available at: http://www.independent.co.uk/news/business/analysis-and-features/is-avandia-set-to-be-glaxos-vioxx-451920.html (Accessed February 19, 2008)

32. Home, PD et al. "Rosiglitazone Evaluated for Cardiovascular Outcomes – An Interim Analysis" New England Journal of Medicine 2007; 357:28-38

33. GlaxoSmithKline Press Release "GlaxoSmithKline to Revise Avandia (Rosiglitazone Maleate) Label in Europe Following Assessment by CHMP" Issued January 24, 2008, London, UK. Available at: http://www.gsk.com/media/pressreleases/2008/2008_pressrelease_0033.htm (Accessed February 19, 2008)

34. The Action to Control Cardiovascular Risk in Diabetes Study Group "Effects of Intensive Glucose Lowering in Type 2 Diabetes" New England Journal of Medicine 2008; 358:2545-2559

35. "GlaxoSmithKline Responds to Findings in ACCORD Study" Issued February 6, 2008, London, UK & Philadelphia, US. Available at: http://www.gsk.com/media/pressreleases/2008/2008_pressrelease_0110.htm (Accessed June 18, 2008)

36.Drazen, JM, Morrissey, S and Curfman, GD "Rosiglitazone – Continued Uncertainty about Safety" New England Journal of Medicine 2007; 357:63-64

37. Wager, E "Authors, Ghosts, Damned Lies, and Statisticians" PLoS Medicine 2007; 4:0005-0006

38. Gotzsche, PC et al. "Ghost Authorship in Industry-Initiated Randomised Trials" PLoS Medicine 2007; 4:0047-0052

39. Gravelle, H, Sutton, M and Ma, A "Doctor Behaviour under a Pay for Performance Contract: Evidence from the Quality and Outcomes Framework" CHE Research Paper 28. University of York and University of Aberdeen. May 2007. Available at: http://www.york.ac.uk/inst/che/pdf/rp28.pdf (Accessed June 19, 2008)

40. Krumholz, HM and Lee, TH "Redefining Quality — Implications of Recent Clinical Trials" New England Journal of Medicine 2008; 358:2537-2539

Chapter 10

1. Mortensen, SA et al. "Dose-Related Decrease of Serum Coenzyme Q10 During Treatment with HMG-CoA Reductase Inhibitors" Molecular Aspects of Medicine 1997; 18 Supplement 1:S137-144

2. Borel, P et al. "Human Plasma Levels of Vitamin E and Carotenoids Are Associated with Genetic Polymorphisms in Genes Involved in Lipid

Metabolism" Journal of Nutrition 2007; 137:2653-2659

3. Packer, L 1993 "Vitamin E In Health and Disease" CRC Press

4. Benowicz, RJ. 1979 "Vitamins and You: A Simple No-Nonsense Guide to the Intelligent Use of Natural and Synthetic Vitamins" Grosset and Dunlap, New York

5. DeCava, JA. 2006 "The Real Truth About Vitamins and Anti-oxidants" 2nd Edition Selene River Press, Fort Collins

6. Colpo, Anthony. 2006 "The Great Cholesterol Con: Why Everything You've Told About Cholesterol, Diet and Heart Disease is Wrong!" www.Lulu.com

7. Barter, PJ et al. "Effects of Torcetrapib in Patients at High Risk for Coronary Events" New England Journal of Medicine 2007; 357:2109-2122

8. Psaty, BM et al. "Potential for Conflict of Interest in the Evaluation of Suspected Adverse Drug Reactions: Use of Cerivastatin and Risk of Rhabdomyolysis" Journal of the American Medical Association 2004; 292:2622-2631

9 Weber, W "Drug Firm Withdraws Statin From the Market" The Lancet 2001; 358(9281):568

10. "FDA Reports More Than Half of Post-Approval Prescription Drug Studies Not Begun" California Healthline May 23, 2003. Available at: http://www.californiahealthline.org/articles/2003/5/23/FDA-Reports-More-Than-Half-of-PostApproval-Prescription-Drug-Studies-Not-Begun.aspx?archive=1 (Accessed 19 December 2007)

11. Ravnskov, U et al. "Should We Lower Cholesterol As Much As Possible?" British Medical Journal 2006; 332:1330-1332

12. Gale, EA. "Lessons from the Glitazones: A Story of Drug Development" The Lancet 2001; 357:1870-1875

13. Horton, R "The Less Acceptable Face of Bias" The Lancet 2000; 356:959-960

14. Kendrick, M. "Should Women be Offered Cholesterol Lowering Drugs to Prevent Cardiovascular Disease? No" British Medical Journal 2007; 334:983

15. Shepherd, J et al. "Pravastatin In Elderly Individuals At Risk of Vascular Disease (PROSPER): A Randomized Controlled Trial" The Lancet 2002; 360:1623-1630

16. Alsheikh-Ali, AA et al. "Effect of the Magnitude of Lipid Lowering on Risk of Elevated Liver Enzymes, Rhabdomyolysis, and Cancer" Journal of the American College of Cardiology 2007; 50:409-418

17. Graveline, D. 2006 "Lipitor Thief of Memory: Statin drugs and the Misguided War on Cholesterol" Duane Graveline www.spacedoc.net

18. Wagstaff LR et al "Statin-Associated Memory Loss: Analysis of 60 Case Reports and Review of the Literature" Pharmacotherapy 2003; 23: 871-880

19. King DS et al. "Cognitive Impairment Associated With Atorvastatin and Simvastatin" Pharmacotherapy 2003; 23: 1663-1667

20. Golomb, BA, Kane, T, Dimsdale, JE. "Severe Irritability Associated With Statin

Cholesterol Lowering" QJM 2004; 97: 229-235

21. Rizvi, K Hampson, JP Harvey, JN. "Do Lipid-Lowering Drugs Cause Erectile Dysfunction? A Systematic Review. Family Practice 2002;19:95-98

22. de Graaf, L et al. "Is Decreased Libido Associated With the Use of HMG-CoA-Reductase Inhibitors?" British Journal of Clinical Pharmacology 2004; 58(3):326-328

23. Edison, RJ and Muenke, M. "Central Nervous System and Limb Anomalies in Case Reports of First-Trimester Statin Exposure" New England Journal of Medicine 2004; 350:1579

24. Tomlinson, SS and Mangione, KK. "Potential Adverse Effects of Statins On Muscle" Physical Therapy 2005; 85(5):459-465

25. Pasternak, RC et al. "ACC/AHA/NHLBI Clinical Advisory On The Use and Safety of Statins" Circulation 2002; 106:1024–1028

26. Ucar, M, Mjorndal, T, Dahlqvist, R. "HMG-CoA Reductase Inhibitors and Myotoxicity" Drug Safety 2000; 22:441–457

27. Cannon, CP et al. "Intensive Versus Moderate Lipid Lowering With Statins After Acute Coronary Syndromes" New England Journal of Medicine 2004; 350:1495–1504

28. Sinzinger, H, Wolfram, R, Peskar, BA. "Muscular Side Effects of Statins" Journal of Cardiovascular Pharmacology 2002; 40:163–171

29. Sinzinger, H, O'Grady, J. "Professional Athletes Suffering From Familial Hypercholesterolaemia Rarely Tolerate Statin Treatment Because of Muscular Problems." British Journal of Clinical Pharmacology 2004; 57:525–528

Chapter 11

1. Crossman, D "Science, Medicine, and the Future: The Future of the Management of Ischaemic Heart Disease" British Medical Journal 1997; 314:356

2. Ross, R "Atherosclerosis – An Inflammatory Disease" New England Journal of Medicine 1999; 340:115-126

3. Ravnskov, Uffe. 2003 "Myth 4: Cholesterol Blocks Arteries" in "The Cholesterol Myths: Exposing the Fallacy that Cholesterol and Saturated Fat Cause Heart Disease" NewTrends, Washington, DC

4. Hansson, GK "Inflammation, Atherosclerosis, and Coronary Artery Disease" New England Journal of Medicine 2005; 352:1685-1695

5. Shishehbor, MH, Bhatt, DL and Topol, EJ "Using C-Reactive Protein to Assess Cardiovascular Disease Risk" Cleveland Clinic Journal of Medicine 2003; 70(7):634-640

6. Ridker, PM "C-Reactive Protein and the Prediction of Cardiovascular Events Among Those at Intermediate Risk: Moving an Inflammatory Hypothesis Toward Consensus" Journal of the American College of Cardiology; 2007;

49:2129-2138

7. Patel, VB, Robbins, MA and Topol, EJ "C-Reactive Protein: A 'Golden Marker' for Inflammation and Coronary Artery Disease" Cleveland Clinic Journal of Medicine 2001; 68(6):521-534

8. Beattie, MS et al "C-Reactive Protein and Ischemia in Users and Nonusers of B-Blockers and Statins: Data From the Heart and Soul Study" Circulation 2003; 107:245-250

9. Chan, AW et al "Relation of Inflammation and Benefit of Statins After Percutaneous Coronary Interventions" Circulation 2003; 107:1750-1756

10. Davignon, J "Beneficial Cardiovascular Pleiotropic Effects of Statins" Circulation 2004; 109[Suppl III];III-39-III-43

11. Schonbeck, U and Libby, P "Inflammation, Immunity, and HMG-CoA Reductase Inhibitors: Statins as Antiinflammatory Agents?" Circulation 2004; 109[Suppl II]:II-18-II-26

12. Packard, CJ et al "Lipoprotein-Associated Phospholipase A2 As An Independent Predictor of Coronary Heart Disease" New England Journal of Medicine 2000; 343:1148-1155

13. Selye, H. 1984 "The Stress of Life" Revised Edition McGraw-Hill

14. Pasceri, V and Yeh, ET "A Tale of Two Diseases: Atherosclerosis and Rheumatoid Arthritis" Circulation. 1999; 100: 2124–2126

15. Wiley, TS and Formby, B. 2000 "Lights Out: Sleep, Sugar and Survival" Pocket Books, New York

16. Braunwald, E "Cardiovascular Medicine at the Turn of the Millennium: Triumphs, Concerns, and Opportunities" New England Journal of Medicine 1997; 337:1360-1369

17. Michiels, C "Endothelial Cell Functions" Journal of Cellular Physiology 2003; 196(3):430 - 443

18. Ridker, PM et al "Comparison of C-Reactive Protein and Low-Density Lipoprotein Cholesterol Levels in the Prediction of First Cardiovascular Events" New England Journal of Medicine 2002; 347:1557-1565

19. Nissen, SE et al "Statin Therapy, LDL Cholesterol, C-Reactive Protein, and Coronary Artery Disease" New England Journal of Medicine 2005; 352:29-38

20. Ridker, PM et al "C-Reactive Protein Levels and Outcomes after Statin Therapy" New England Journal of Medicine 2005; 352:20-28

21. Yeh, ET, Willerson, JT "Coming of Age of C-Reactive Protein: Using Inflammation Markers in Cardiology" Circulation 2003; 107:370-371

22. Balk, EM et al. "Effects of Statins on Nonlipid serum Markers Associated with Cardiovascular Disease: A Systematic Review" Annals of Internal Medicine 2003; 139:670-682

23. Ridker, PM et al. "Inflammation, Pravastatin, and the Risk of Coronary Events After Myocardial Infarction in Patients With Average Cholesterol Levels"

Circulation 1998; 98:839-844

24. Gurm, H and Hoogwerf, B "The Heart Protection Study: High-Risk Patients Benefit from Statins, Regardless of LDL-C Level" Cleveland Clinic Journal of Medicine 2003; 70(11):991-997

25. Heart Protection Study Collaborative Group "MRC/BHF Heart Protection Study of Cholesterol Lowering With Simvastatin in 20,536 High-Risk Individuals: A Randomised Placebo-Controlled Trial" Lancet 2002; 360:7–22

26. Ravnskov, U "Conclusions from the Heart Protection Study were Premature" British Medical Journal 2002; 324:789

27. Plenge, JK et al. "Simvastatin Lowers C-Reactive Protein Within 14 Days: An Effect Independent of Low-Density Lipoprotein Cholesterol Reduction" Circulation 2002; 106:1447-1452

28. McCarey, DW et al "Trial of Atorvastatin in Rheumatoid Arthritis (TARA): Double-Blind, Randomised Placebo-Controlled Trial" Lancet 2004; 363:2015-2021

29. McCully, KS and McCully, M. 2000 "The Heart Revolution: The Extraordinary Discovery That Finally Laid the Cholesterol Myth to Rest" HarperPerennial, New York

30. Hackam, DG and Anand, SS "Emerging Risk Factors for Atherosclerotic Vascular Disease: A Critical Review of the Evidence" Journal of the American Medical Association 2003; 290:932-940

31. Wald,DS, Law,M and Morris, JK "Homocysteine and Cardiovascular Disease: Evidence on Causality from a Meta-Analysis" British Medical Journal 2002; 325: 1202 – 1206

32. Selhub, J et al "Vitamin Status and Intake As Primary Determinants of Homocysteinemia in an Elderly Population" Journal of the American Medical Association 1993; 270:2693-2698

Chapter 12

1. Stumvoll, M, Goldstein, BJ, and van Haeften, TW "Type 2 Diabetes: Principles of Pathogenesis and Therapy" Lancet 2005; 365:1333-1346

2. Heine, RJ et al. "Management of Hyperglycaemia in Type 2 Diabetes" British Medical Journal 2006; 333:1200-1204

3. Diabetes UK Webpage "Myths" Available at: http://www.diabetes.org.uk/Guide-to-diabetes/What_is_diabetes/Myths/ (Accessed April 15, 2008)

4. Diabetes UK Webpage "Causes and Risk Factors" Available at: http://www.diabetes.org.uk/Guide-to-diabetes/What_is_diabetes/Causes_and_Risk_Factors/ (Accessed April 15, 2008)

5. Diabetes UK Webpage "Treating Diabetes" Available at: http://www.diabetes.org.uk/Guide-to-diabetes/What_is_diabetes/Treating_diabetes/ (Accessed April 15, 2008)

6. Haslam, DW and James, WPT "Obesity" Lancet 2005; 366:1197-1209

7. Diabetes UK Webpage "Balancing Your Diet" Available at: http://www.diabetes.org.uk/Guide-to-diabetes/Food_and_recipes/Food_and_diabetes/Balancing_your_diet/ (Accessed April 15, 2008)

8. Colhoun, HM et al. "Primary Prevention of Cardiovascular Disease with Atorvastatin in Type 2 Diabetes in the Collaborative Atorvastatin Diabetes Study (CARDS): Multicentre Randomised Placebo-Controlled Trial" Lancet 2004; 364:685-696

9. Sniderman, AD et al. "Hypertriglyceridemic HyperapoB in Type 2 Diabetes" Diabetes Care 2002; 25:579-582

10. "Prevalence of Risk Factors for CVD in People with Diabetes" Chapter 4 of the British Heart Foundation Coronary Heart Disease Statistics: Diabetes Supplement. 2001 Edition. Available at: http://www.heartstats.org/datapage.asp?id=3258

11. Liu, S et al. "Dietary Glycemic Load assessed by Food-Frequency Questionnaire in Relation to Plasma High-Density-Lipoprotein Cholesterol and Fasting Plasma Triacylglycerols in Postmenopausal Women" American Journal of Clinical Nutrition 2001;73:560-566

12. Radhika, G et al. "Dietary Carbohydrates, Glycemic Load and Serum High-Density Lipoprotein Cholesterol Concentrations among South Indian Adults" European Journal of Clinical Nutrition. Advance Online Publication November 7, 2007

13. Garg, A, Grundy, SM and Koffler, M "Effect of High Carbohydrate Intake on Hyperglycemia, Islet Function, and Plasma Lipoproteins in NIDDM" Diabetes Care 1992; 15:1572-1580

14. Garg, A et al. "Effects of Varying Carbohydrate Content of Diet in Patients with Non-Insulin-Dependent Diabetes Mellitus" Journal of the American Medical Association 1994; 271:1421-1428

15. Samaha, FF et al. "A Low-Carbohydrate as Compared with a Low-Fat Diet in Severe Obesity" New England Journal of Medicine 2003; 348:2074-2081

16. Yancy, WS et al. "A Low-Carbohydrate, Ketogenic Diet Verses a Low-Fat Diet to Treat Obesity and Hyperlipidemia". Annals of Internal Medicine 2004; 140:769-777

17. Gardner, CD et al. "Comparison of the Atkins, Zone, Ornish and LEARN Diets for Change in Weight and Related Risk Factors among Overweight Premenopausal Women". Journal of the American Medical Association 2007; 297:969-977

18. Stern, L et al. "The Effects of Low-Carbohydrate Verses Conventional Weight Loss Diets in Severely Obese Adults: One-Year Follow-up of a Randomized Trial". Annals of Internal Medicine 2004; 140:778-785

19. Foster, GD et al. "A Randomized Trial of a Low-Carbohydrate Diet for

REFERENCES

Obesity" New England Journal of Medicine 2003; 348:2082-2090

20. Appel. LJ et al. "Effects of Protein, Monounsaturated Fat, and Carbohydrate Intake on Blood Pressure and Serum Lipids" Journal of the American Medical Association 2005; 294: 2455-2464

21. Mozaffarian, D, Rimm, EB, and Herrington, DM "Dietary Fats, Carbohydrate, and Progression of Coronary Atherosclerosis in Postmenopausal Women" American Journal of Clinical Nutrition 2004; 80:1175-1184

22. Beckman, JA, Creager, MA, and Libby, P "Diabetes and Atherosclerosis: Epidemiology, Pathophysiology, and Management" Journal of the American Medical Association 2002; 287:2570-2581

23. Syvanne, M and Taskinen, M "Lipids and Lipoproteins as Coronary Risk Factors in Non-Insulin Dependent Diabetes Mellitus" Lancet 1997; 350(suppl l):20-23

24. Sniderman, AD, Scantlebury, T and Cianflone, K "Hypertriglyceridemic HyperapoB: The Unappreciated Atherogenic Dyslipoproteinemia in Type 2 Diabetes Mellitus" Annals of Internal Medicine 2001; 135:447-459

25. Zhengling, Li et al. "Men and Women Differ in Lipoprotein Response to Dietary Saturated Fat and Cholesterol Restriction" Journal of Nutrition 2003; 133:3428-3433

26. Walden, CE et al. "Lipoprotein Lipid Response to the National Cholesterol Education Program Step II Diet by Hypercholesterolemic and Combined Hyperlipidemic Women and Men" Arteriosclerosis, Thrombosis, and Vascular Biology 1997;17:375-382

27. Lichtenstein, AH et al. "Efficacy of a Therapeutic Lifestyle Change/Step 2 Diet in Moderately Hypercholesterolemic Middle-Aged and Elderly Female and Male Subjects" Journal of Lipid Research 2002; 43:264-273

28. Barzilai, N et al. "Unique Lipoprotein Phenotype and Genotype Associated With Exceptional Longevity" Journal of the American Medical Association 2003; 290:2030-2040

29. Coresh, J et al "Association of Plasma Triglyceride Concentration and LDL Particle Diameter, Density, and Chemical Composition with Premature Coronary Artery Disease in Men and Women" Journal of Lipid Research 1993; 34:1687-1697

30. Campos, H et al. "Low Density Lipoprotein Particle Size and Coronary Artery Disease" Arteriosclerosis, Thrombosis, and Vascular Biology 1992; 12:187-195

31. Heijmans, BT et al. "Lipoprotein Particle Profiles Mark Familial and Sporadic Human Longevity" PLoS Medicine 2006; 3(12):2317-2323

32. Dreon, DM et al. "Change in Dietary Saturated Fat Intake is Correlated with Change in Mass of Large Low-Density-Lipoprotein Particles in Men" American Journal of Clinical Nutrition 1998; 67:828-836

33. Sjogren, P et al. "Milk-Derived Fatty Acids Are Associated with a More

Favourable LDL Particle Size Distribution in Healthy Men" Journal of Nutrition 2004; 134:1729-1735

34. Dreon, DM et al. "Reduced LDL Particle Size in Children Consuming a Very-Low-Fat Diet is Related to Parental LDL-Subclass Patterns" American Journal of Clinical Nutrition 2000; 71(6):1611-1616

35. Dreon, DM et al. "A Very-Low-Fat Diet is Not Associated With Improved Lipoprotein Profiles in Men With a Predominance of Large, Low-Density Lipoproteins" American Journal of Clinical Nutrition 1999; 69:411-418

36. Kim, MK and Campos, H "Intake of Trans Fatty Acids and Low-Density Lipoprotein Size in a Costa Rican Population" Metabolism 2003; 52(6):693-698

37. Webster, MW and Scott, RS "What Cardiologists Need to Know about Diabetes" Lancet 1997; 350 Suppl 1:SI23- SI28

38. Beckman, JA, Creager, MA and Libby, P "Diabetes and Atherosclerosis: Epidemiology, Pathophysiology, and Management" Journal of the American Medical Association 2002; 287:2570-2581

39. Ludwig, DS "The Glycemic Index: Physiological Mechanisms Relating to Obesity, Diabetes, and Cardiovascular Disease" Journal of the American Medical Association 2002; 287:2414-2423

40. Williams, SB et al. "Acute Hyperglycemia Attenuates Endothelium-Dependent Vasodilation in Humans In Vivo" Circulation 1998; 97:1695-1701

41. Title, LM et al. "Oral Glucose Loading Acutely Attenuates Endothelium-Dependent Vasodilation in Healthy Adults Without Diabetes: An Effect Prevented by Vitamins C and E" Journal of the American College of Cardiology 2000;36:2185-2191

42. Williams, SB et al. "Impaired Nitric Oxide-Mediated Vasodilation in Patients with Non-Insulin-Dependent Diabetes Mellitus" Journal of the American College of Cardiology 1996;27:567-574

43. Coutinho, M et al. "The Relationship between Glucose and Incident Cardiovascular Events. A Metaregression Analysis of Published Data from 20 Studies of 95,783 Individuals Followed for 12.4 Years" Diabetes Care 1999; 22:233-240

44. "Diabetes" Chapter 12 of the British Heart Foundation Coronary Heart Disease Statistics. July 2007 Available at: http://www.heartstats.org/datapage.asp?id=6799 (Accessed April 16, 2008)

45. Packer, L 1993 "Vitamin E In Health and Disease" CRC Press

46. Liu, S et al. "Relation between a Diet with a High Glycemic Load and Plasma Concentrations of High-Sensitivity C-Reactive Protein in Middle-Aged Women" American Journal of Clinical Nutrition 2002; 75:492-498

47. Shai, I et al. "Weight Loss with a Low-Carbohydrate, Mediterranean, or Low-Fat Diet" New England Journal of Medicine 2008; 359:229-241

48. Rapaport, L "Bristol-Myers' New-Type Diabetes Drug Controls Sugar, Weight"

Bloomberg.com June 7, 2008. Available at: http://www.bloomberg.com/ apps/news?pid=20601087&sid=aNWJdyfsrApE&refer=home (Accessed July 6, 2008)

49. Berkrot, B "Bristol Diabetes Drug Effective, Safe, Study Shows" Reuters June 7, 2008. Available at: http://www.reuters.com/article/healthNews/ idUSN0637255720080607 (Accessed July 6, 2008)

50. "Amylin Shares Recover on Diabetes Drug Data" Associated Press June 10, 2008 Available at: http://www.forbes.com/feeds/ap/2008/06/10/ ap5102042.html (Accessed July 6, 2008)

Chapter 13

1. Hawkes, N "The Pill of Life that Keeps on Working" The Times Newspaper, October 11, 2007

2. Downs, JR et al. "Primary Prevention of Acute Coronary Events with Lovastatin in Men and Women with Average Cholesterol Levels: Results of AFCAPS/TexCAPS" Journal of the American Medical Association 1998; 279:1615-1622

3. Sever, PS et al. "Prevention of Coronary and Stroke Events with Atorvastatin in Hypertensive Patients who have Average or Lower-Than-Average Cholesterol Concentrations, in the Anglo-Scandinavian Cardiac Outcomes Trial—Lipid Lowering Arm (ASCOT-LLA): A Multicentre Randomised Controlled Trial" Lancet 2003; 361:1149-1158

4. Cholesterol Treatment Trialists' (CTT) Collaborators "Efficacy and Safety of Cholesterol-Lowering Treatment: Prospective Meta-Analysis of Data from 90,056 Participants in 14 Randomised Trials of Statins" Lancet 2005; 366:1267-1278

5. Cholesterol Treatment Trialists' (CTT) Collaborators "Efficacy of Cholesterol-Lowering Therapy in 18686 People with Diabetes in 14 Randomised Trials of Statins: A Meta-Analysis" Lancet 2008; 371:117-125

6. Heart Protection Study Collaborative Group "MRC/BHF Heart Protection Study of Cholesterol Lowering with Simvastatin in 20,536 High-Risk Individuals: A Randomised Placebo-Controlled Trial" Lancet 2002; 360:7-22

7. No authors listed "Randomised Trial of Cholesterol Lowering in 4444 Patients with Coronary Heart Disease: the Scandinavian Simvastatin Survival Study (4S)" Lancet 1994; 344:1383-1389

8. Deedwania, P et al. "Reduction of Low-Density Lipoprotein Cholesterol in Patients with Coronary Heart Disease and Metabolic Syndrome: Analysis of the Treating to New Targets Study" Lancet 2006; 368:919-928

9. Shepherd, J et al. "Prevention of Coronary Heart Disease with Pravastatin in Men with Hypercholesterolemia" New England Journal of Medicine 1995; 333:1301-1308

10. British Heart Foundation "All About Statins" Available at: http://www.bhf.org.uk/living_with_heart_conditions/treatment/medicines_for_the_heart/statins.aspx (Accessed April 14, 2008)

11. Samani, NJ and de Bono, DP "Prevention of Coronary Heart Disease with Pravastatin" New England Journal of Medicine, Correspondence 1996; 334:1333-1335

12. "Smoking" Chapter 4 of the British Heart Foundation Coronary Heart Disease Statistics. July 2007 Available at: http://www.heartstats.org/datapage.asp?id=6799 (Accessed April 14, 2007)

13. Bakhru, A and Erlinger, TP "Smoking Cessation and Cardiovascular Disease Risk Factors: Results from the Third National Health and Nutrition Examination Survey" PloS Medicine 2005; 2:0528-0536

14. Ford, I et al. "Long-Term Follow-Up of the West of Scotland Coronary Prevention Study" New England Journal of Medicine 2007; 357:1477-1486

15. Domanski, MJ "Primary Prevention of Coronary Artery Disease" New England Journal of Medicine 2007; 357:1543-1545

Chapter 14

1. "Lower Cholesterol the Easy Way" Information published on the Unilever website about Flora pro.activ. Available at: http://www.unilever.co.uk/ourbrands/casestudies/floraproactive_casestudy.asp (Accessed April 26, 2008)

2. Starling, S "UK Sterol Foods Market Slows Amid Consumer Confusion" NutraIncredients.com March 27, 2008 Available at: http://www.nutraingredients.com/news/ng.asp?id=84254-pro-activ-benecol-probiotics-sterols-cholesterol-lowering (Accessed April 27, 2008)

3. Smith, R "Don't Bother with Foods that Lower Cholesterol" Telegraph Newspaper May 31, 2008 Available at: http://www.telegraph.co.uk/news/uknews/2055339/National-Institute-for-Health-and-Clinical-Excellence-advise-patients-not-to-bother-with-foods-that-lower-cholesterol.html (Accessed August 14, 2008)

4. Erasmus, U 1993 "Fats That Heal Fats That Kill" Alive Books, Canada

5. Campbell-McBride, N 2004 "Gut and Psychology Syndrome" Mediform Publishing, Cambridge, UK

6. Blaylock, RL 1997 "Excitotoxins: The Taste that Kills" Health Press, New Mexico

7. Mozaffarian, D et al. "Trans Fatty Acids and Cardiovascular Disease" New England Journal of Medicine 2006; 354:1601-1613

8. Information published by Unilever on their Flora pro.activ website. "How is Flora Made" Available at: http://www.florapro-activ.com.au/245_250.htm (Accessed April 27, 2008)

9. Mauger, J et al. "Effect of Different Forms of Dietary Hydrogenated Fats on LDL Particle Size" American Journal of Clinical Nutrition 2003; 78:370-375

10. Patel, S "Dietary Cholesterol Absorption" Lancet 2001; 358:s63

11. Law, M "Plant Sterol and Stanol Margarines and Health" British Medical Journal 2000; 320:861-864

12. Thurnham, DI "Functional Foods: Cholesterol-Lowering Benefits of Plant Sterols" British Journal of Nutrition 1999; 82:255-256

13. Cleghorn, CL et al. "Plant Sterol-Enriched Spread Enhances the Cholesterol-Lowering Potential of a Fat-Reduced Diet" European Journal of Clinical Nutrition 2003; 57:170-176

14. Scientific Committee on Food 2003 "Opinion of the Scientific Committee on Food on an Application from ADM for Approval of Plant Sterol-Enriched Foods" European Commission, Brussels. SCF/CS/NF/DOS/23 ADD2 Final. April 7, 2003

15. Davidson, MH et al. "Safety and Tolerability of Esterified Phytosterols Administered in Reduced-Fat Spread and Salad Dressing to Healthy Adult Men and Women" Journal of the American College of Nutrition 2001; 20:307-319

16. DeCava, JA. 2006 "The Real Truth About Vitamins and Anti-oxidants" 2nd Edition Selene River Press, Fort Collins

17. Noakes, M et al. "An Increase in Dietary Carotenoids When Consuming Plant Sterols or Stanols is Effective in Maintaining Plasma Carotenoid Concentrations" American Journal of Clinical Nutrition 2002; 75:79-86

18. Simopoulos, AP "The Importance of the Ratio of Omega-6/Omega-3 Essential Fatty Acids" Biomedicine and Pharmacotherapy 2002; 56:365-379

19. Fallon, S and Enig, M. 2001 "Nourishing Traditions: The Cookbook that Challenges Politically Correct Nutrition and the Diet Dictocrats" NewTrends, Washington DC

INDEX